DEDICATION

To have written three books, this being the third, gives me such massive joy, particularly as my mother was a librarian for most of her life and instilled in me the importance of books.

She was a librarian when she met my dad and when they got married he encouraged her to give up work as her income wasn't required but it was only until Mummy Bear had me, that she surrendered and gave up her position as librarian at Monsanto's - a place she has never stopped talking about.

As soon as my sister was old enough, Mummy Bear got another job as a librarian at a local High School, Hartridge, where, let's just say the pupils can be quite interesting!

Her enthusiasm for books was absolutely magnificent, which was how in a troubled school she managed to get so many engaged and took so much pride in her library. I used to pop in most weeks to see her during the day and it brings tears to my eyes as I write this, going back in time and recalling how happy she was in that environment.

When she was made redundant it absolutely broke her heart. She fought for her job, however it was not to be…

Sadly my mother has not been able to see that her son has written these books, since though she is still alive, she has final stages of dementia. This means that, no matter how many times I show her, just a few moments later she loses the memory. I however, retain the knowledge that in those few moments I can see how proud she is.

I do wonder if without Mummy Bear's magical enthusiasm and charm, would I have read so many books with such gusto and spent the many years writing these books whilst peers are off making bucket loads of money...?

I am most truly blessed and humbled to have such a great mother.

STOP!! Waking Up Tired...

The Beginners Guide to Sleep

RALPH MONTAGUE

Published: March 2023 by FCM Publishing
ISBN 978-1-914529-62-7 - Paperback
ISBN 978-1-914529-63-4 - eBook

This book is intended as a reference volume only, not as a medical manual. The information given here is designed to help you make informed decisions about your health. It is not intended as any substitute for any treatment that may have been prescribed by your doctor. If you suspect that you have a medical problem, we urge you to seek medical help.

Praise for the STOP!! Workbook series

"Informative life lessons with a dash of humour"

- Gareth Cooper British Lion

"A thought-provoking life - changer!"

- Leigh Beddington
British Judo Champion

"Practical and humorous advice. A life-enhancing workbook"

- Ray Star Award-winning Author

"Entertaining. Easy to follow. A compelling read to help you take control of your life"

- Patti Diener Podcast Host

"A guardian angel on my shoulder!"

-Thomas Bryan
Independent review

ACKNOWLEDGEMENTS

Two people in particular spring to mind when it comes to getting this book ship shape and Bristol fashion.

My publicist Tina Higginson of FCM Media - we have such a great laugh together and speak pretty much every day. It's been a real pleasure working with her and makes this work of mine, such a delight. So, a massive thankyou Tina!

Next is my publisher, Taryn Johnston, at FCM Publishing, who will send me very provoking edits back, really questioning statements I have made. We've certainly had some interesting discussions around comparing sugar and heroin on my last book STOP!! Killing Yourself…The Beginners Guide to Living Longer.

Without Tina, no one would know my books even exist, except for my mum and dad!

Without Taryn, this book wouldn't have been released for some time, if at all and these books would not be of the high-quality and standard that they are.

TABLE OF CONTENTS

"Tomorrow Starts the Night Before…"

— Me!

GETTING STARTED...
SLEEPING BETTER STARTS HERE!

WHY I WROTE THIS BOOK 1

I could not have written this chapter at a more appropriate time, having experienced the after effects of alcohol over the weekend and the hugely destructive role it has played in my sleep the last few nights.

When I don't sleep well, I don't live well, both emotionally and energetically. I miss that feeling of simply feeling good in myself. The high level of energy and motivation to get things done with enthusiasm and a smile on my face.

That every morning feeling where you, "beat the alarm clock" as I like to call it. Where you are so revved up to go, you simply cannot wait any longer for the alarm clock to go off as you just want to get up now and hit the day running – well, sprinting…

It is for those reasons I wrote this book and like my first book in the STOP!! Series this started out as a guide for me to fully optimise tomorrow, the night before.

In fact in STOP!! Killing Yourself I have an entire chapter on sleep, due to its importance on living longer, however I have since realised that just one chapter is not enough. It needed an entire book, just on this one subject alone. Though the chapter is a great introduction for those looking to sleep better, I really wanted to take things to the next level, so you are in for a treat now.

Sleep is the most important daily activity that you and I as humans undertake. I go into the facts in the next chapter however, here it's more to describe the emotional and non-tangibles.

I was dating someone recently who found it hard to lie next to someone in silence. Ironically if she had stopped worrying about being in silence, she would be in silence and even more importantly unaware! She would get up around 2am, to either sleep on the sofa or book a taxi and go home.

Why do I tell you this? Well, one of the reasons for us splitting up and me not wanting to continue the relationship, was that it was significantly affecting my work. The beautiful irony was that this book ended up being a few weeks late due to me not sleeping well!

After spending the night (well half the night!) with her and then being awakened at 2am, I would find that the next day I would now be operating at a level of indifference that drove me mad! I would sit at my desk unmotivated and know what I did eventually write was substandard and therefore in turn was pointless, so I would simply sit on the sofa unproductive and frustrated!

There is nothing better than come wakey-wakey time, you simply leap out of bed with no alarm clock, are super excited and in fact chomping at the bit to get out of bed! Just ask my supportive and beautiful ex-fiancé of many years, who had to endure the daily torture of being abruptly awoken at 5.30am every morning, with a wild, crazy and rather loud man wanting to discuss business and plans, all while dancing excitedly around the bedroom. She was not impressed, but I'm sure deep down she appreciated the enthusiasm in which her day started...

When I do my normal days, utilising everything that I have learned, researched and tested over the last twenty years, the level I operate is like comparing driving a BMX to an Aston Martin and I've had both.

I am sure that I am not alone in needing better sleep, and it's for this reason I share my insights, experiences, experiments, failings and triumphs in this book, so you don't have to.

It's not often I would say this about my books however, I really do hope this book sends you to sleep…

"I think it is good that books still exist,
but they do make me sleepy."

— Frank Zappa, The Real Frank Zappa Book

WHY IS SLEEP THE MOST IMPORTANT THING IN YOUR LIFE?

2

Increase Your Risk of Heart Attacks

Sleeping fewer than seven hours every night, increases your risk of heart disease by 13%, which is unlucky for some it would seem.

Did you know that by sleeping as little as just five hours each night as opposed to seven, you increase your risk of high blood pressure by a whopping 61%!

Fancy Diabetes?

Well one of the best ways after eating lots of sugar to do this, is simply by sleeping less! Yes, it's that easy for those "dying" to get diabetes…

By only sleeping five hours each night you increase your chances of getting diabetes by almost 50%.

By sleeping less, you are interfering with your body's ability to regulate insulin, reducing its sensitivity.

Your Body's Immune System

Without sleep your immune system cannot function properly. It's that simple.

Simple everyday issues like say catching a cold, are increased almost five-fold for those who sleep less than five hours a night.

If it's having this effect on an everyday cold, can you imagine what's happening to more serious things going on in your body?

Helps Prevent Being Overweight

Sleep helps maintain your natural and healthy body weight i.e. not overweight! If you are getting less than seven hours of sleep each night, you have a 41% increased chance of being obese.

Sleep deprivation increases levels of your hormone ghrelin that makes us feel hungry, while simultaneously reducing our leptin levels which makes us feel full. So, a double whammy here...

Which is why you will find those who are sleep deprived, also eat the most! And it's not because they are greedy or glutinous, the common belief people have. They also abuse their consumption of artificial stimulants such as sugar, energy drinks and caffeine (which is natural).

Plus, we all know that when feeling tired we are less likely to exercise, in turn creating a snowballing effect.

Improve Your Productivity and Concentration Levels

If you want to be successful, then you need a few key brain functions to achieve this, such as:

- Productivity.
- Concentration.
- Cognitive abilities.

Just by sleeping less, you can double the amount of work-related errors that you make - yes double! Imagine making twice the number of mistakes every day, simply because you haven't slept enough.

Problem solving skills are also boosted by a great night's sleep!

Feeling Depressed or Anxious?

It's not just full-blown depression that's linked to poor sleep, it's all types of mental health, however depression is certainly the icing on the cake when you don't take your sleep seriously.

Anxiety, which can be crippling for some, is also massively increased when you don't get a good night's sleep.

Sleep plays such a key role in the regulation of our central nervous system. Which in turn manages our response to stress, the fight or flight in us!

It's these bodily systems (sympathetic nervous system and HPA axis) that regulate our inflammatory signalling pathways. Increased, and more importantly regular, activation of these pathways creates chronic inflammation, the cause of all the world's most popular diseases! Things such as cancer, Alzheimer's, diabetes, heart disease etc., all the pleasant ways to die early!

Are You an Emotional Wreck?

The same reasons why you get stressed easier and more frequently are down to your reduced ability to manage emotions and thoughts from sleep deprivation (classed as under seven hours sleep).

Think to yourself the last time you lost your temper or had some emotional outburst? Were you tired at the time?

Most likely you were, even if you can't remember!

Other emotional aspects that lack of sleep can have, include less serious issues, though nonetheless welcome, such as lack of empathy for others, withdrawing from social interactions and general relationship building with others.

Are You Accident Prone?

We've already covered how sleep effects concentration, errors and focus, however when you start to put this in the context of simple everyday things like driving, you are now exposing yourself to a much higher risk of crashing your car and causing injury or death to yourself and others.

Studies have shown that being sleep deprived is very similar to the effects of alcohol. So by being tired and driving you put yourself at risk of the same dangers to drink driving.

Sleeping less than five hours a night, can double your risk of a car accident, studies have shown. It's that serious! And for those who've slept less than four hours, well, you now have a fifteen times increased chance of a car accident.

"*When you lie down, you will not be afraid.
Your sleep will be sweet.*"

— Proverbs

RALPH'S TOP 10... 3

I f there is a chance you are going to ignore everything else that I cover, then at least pay attention to the following list.

These are big ones; this is like going into a knife fight with a gun.

1. **Consistency**

   Go to bed and wake up at the same time every day. This is one of the most important lessons to learn for a healthier and longer life.

2. **Eat Early**

   Eating late at night and expecting to sleep well, is like drinking ten pints of lager and expecting to still walk in a straight line AND wakeup with no hangover!

3. **Calm Your Mind**

   A busy mind will stop you from sleeping. If your mind is that stressed or active, it could mean in worst cases not getting any sleep at night. Meditation is one of the best ways to become a calmer more relaxed human.

4. **Natural Light**

Get this daily as this is key to setting a well-functioning circadian rhythm (I explain this later) for you.

5. **Exercise**

Is one of the quickest and easiest ways to make you tired, in turn falling asleep quicker and giving you a deeper sleep. Though please leave a few hours between exercise and sleep if possible.

6. **Stimulants**

Stop consuming caffeine, energy drinks or other stimulants after noon ideally, but a hard cut off at 2pm to get a great night's sleep.

7. **Late Night Liquids**

Fed up with waking up during the night for a loo break, which breaks your deep sleep; then lying awake at 3am unable to get back to sleep? Simply stop consuming liquids after 5pm.

8. **A Cool Bedroom**

Will help you fall asleep quicker and give you a deeper sleep.

9. **A Dark Bedroom**

Don't let external light sources keep you stimulated and awake at night.

10. **Ditch Blue Lights**

Mobile phones, tablets and laptops blast you with a type of light that wakes you up just at the time you don't want to be kept up!

If you are one of those highly emotional and reactive types, just by doing one or two of the above you will find life brings you less tears, less tantrums and people will like you more! Plus you never know, now your partner might even want to have sex with you…

"Never waste any time you can spend sleeping."

— Frank H. Knight

HOW LONG SHOULD YOU SLEEP FOR? 4

The quick answer… it depends!

"Well, Ralph, that was really helpful, and I am really glad I came to you for help!"

What About My "Eight Hours" A Night Sleep?

It's worth noting at this point about the old "eight hours a night" parable, QUALITY of sleep is more important than QUANTITY of sleep.

I would rather sleep for just seven hours and get three or four hours of deep sleep and rapid eye movement (REM) than sleep for nine hours and get just two hours of deep sleep and REM.

That being said, guess what the best amount of sleep time is for me… eight hours.

When I sleep for seven hours, which I have experimented with, I don't feel quite as energised and raring to go as when I sleep for eight.

Everyone has a different optimal sleep duration. You will need to experiment a little to find out what yours is, which will be between seven to nine hours; however, this will be somewhere around the eight-hour mark for most. Though please remember everyone is different.

For me, by waking up half an hour earlier and having seven-and-a-half hours of sleep instead of my typical eight hours, I in turn miss out on that extra REM. So, by adding an extra 30 minutes to my sleep, I get an extra 25-30 minutes of REM per night. A price worth paying for getting up half an hour later.

What's the Right Amount of Sleep for You?

Well, it's quite straightforward what you are to do...

For the first few nights, don't set your alarm; just wake up when your body wants to.

"Yes, Ralph, that's all very well for you, but I got kids, I got work...!!"

Ok, so ask yourself, what's more important?

You go into work for a few days at a different time than normal yet now wake up every day full of energy and able to do a high-quality workday for the rest of your life.

Or scraping by as you currently are, waking up feeling like shit? Not fulfilling your full potential and continuously being mentally vacant with your loved ones, as you have run out of energy come the evening (though, let's be honest, you didn't have much to begin with), never mind the health ticking time bomb waiting to blow up inside you.

So, for the next three to four nights, simply wake up when you want.

If you have children or someone you care for that makes this a non-possibility, ask yourself, what can you do to make this a possibility? Is there a friend or relative that can stay around one weekend so that you can gain some perspective on your natural sleeping pattern? Again, I cannot stress this enough, sleep is vital in achieving a healthy, happy lifestyle, so ask that favour, try and make this happen, you owe it to yourself to get your sleep back on track.

If you have to let others know of this, to make this as easy as possible, please do so, as we want your utmost focus on this matter.

It's also worth noting that once you have done this, perhaps suggest that your partner does the same to optimise their sleep as well. This way you are both then operating at your best and in turn can be there for each other in a more present and emotional stable manner.

After a few days of doing this, once you have removed your continuous tiredness every morning (we don't really catch up on sleep longer than a few days however, for ease, to say you have now caught up on your sleep, is a good simple way of conveying this). You may find, after the first morning or two, you sleep for quite a few hours extra. This is fine. Then once you get this out of your system, you will notice a time you like to wake up.

Keep note of this, as you now know how much time your body likes to sleep. From here, you can then plan the time you would like to wake up and, in turn, plan backwards, to determine the time you need to go to bed to facilitate this.

Your Next Steps to a Great Night's Sleep...

Go to sleep for the next three to four nights with no alarm set and see how long your body wants you to sleep without any outside distractions.

Inform people of your plan and perhaps also sleep in a separate bedroom if this further helps.

It's widely known that seven hours is the absolute minimum for nearly all humans, so anything below this will most likely bring you negative health issues in the future. The same goes for too much sleep, which is generally held to be around nine hours. So, your sweet spot will lie somewhere within this range.

"Sleep is the best meditation."

— Dalai Lama

YOUR CHRONOTYPE FACT FIND 5

Before we go straight into my Sleep Coaching model; RIO, (Remove, Improve and Optimise). It's key to understand what chronotype you are.

A chronotype relates to your sleep preferences and plays a huge role in what time you should sleep, how long you sleep, what time you wake up and how you should structure your day for optimum efficiency.

So, we are going to do a test, to see which chronotype you are, from there we can better advise on the best sleep habits for you.

1. **The slightest sound or light keeps you awake or wakes you**
   True or False?

2. **Food is not a great passion for you**
   True or False?

3. **You usually wake up before your alarm**
   True or False?

4. **You don't sleep well on planes, even when you wear an eye mask and earplugs**
   True or False?

5. **You are often irritable due to fatigue**
   True or False?

6. **You worry a lot about small details**
   True or False?

7. **You have been diagnosed by a doctor or self-diagnosed as an insomniac**
   True or False?

8. **You were anxious about your grades in school**
   True or False?

9. **You often lose sleep worrying about what happened in the past and what may happen to you in the future**
   True or False?

10. **You are a perfectionist**
    True or False?

If seven or more are answered TRUE

You are a DOLPHIN.

There is no need to do the rest of this fact find.

1. **If you had nothing to do the next day and gave yourself permission to sleep as long as you like, when would you wake up?**

   a. Before 06:30 - (1).
   b. Between 0630 and 08:45 - (2).
   c. After 08:45 - (3).

2. **When you have to get out of bed by a certain time, do you use an alarm clock?**

   a. No need. You wake up on your own at just the right time - (1).
   b. Yes, to the alarm with no snooze or one snooze - (2).
   c. Yes, to the alarm, with a backup alarm and multiple snoozes - (3).

3. **When do you wake up on the weekends?**

   a. The same time as your work week schedule - (1).
   b. Within 45 mins to 90 mins of your workweek schedule - (2).
   c. 90 mins or more past your workweek schedule - (3).

4. **How do you experience jet lag?**

   a. You struggle with it, no matter what - (1).
   b. You adjust within 48 hours - (2).
   c. You adjust quickly, especially when travelling west - (3).

5. **What's your favourite meal? (Think more time of day than the menu!)**

   a. Breakfast - (1).
   b. Lunch - (2).
   c. Dinner - (3).

6. **If you were to flash back to high school and take your GCSEs again, when would you prefer to start the exam for maximum focus and concentration (not to just get it over with)?**

   a. Early morning - (1).
   b. Early afternoon - (2).
   c. Mid-afternoon - (3).

7. **If you could choose any time of the day to do an intense workout, when would you do it?**

   a. Before 08:00 - (1).
   b. Between 08:00 and 16:00 - (2).
   c. After 16:00 - (3).

8. **When are you most alert?**

   a. One or two hours post wakeup - (1).
   b. Two to four hours post wakeup - (2).
   c. Four to six hours post wakeup - (3).

9. **If you could choose your own five-hour workday, which block of hours would you choose?**

   a. 04:00 to 09:00 - (1).
   b. 09:00 to 14:00 - (2).
   c. 16:00 to 21:00 - (3).

10. **Do you consider yourself?**

   a. Left brained - that is strategic and analytical thinker - (1).
   b. A balanced thinker - (2).
   c. Right brained - that is creative and insightful thinker - (3).

11. Do you nap?

    a.   Never - (1).

    b.   Sometimes on the weekend - (2).

    c.   If you took a nap, you'd be up all night - (3).

12. If you had to do two hours of hard physical labour, like moving furniture or chopping wood, when would you choose to do it for maximum efficiency and safety (not just to get it over with)?

    a.   08:00 to 10:00 – (1).

    b.   11:00 to 13:00 - (2).

    c.   18:00 to 20:00 - (3).

13. Regarding your overall health, which statement sounds like you?

    a.   I make healthy choices almost all the time - (1).

    b.   I make healthy choices sometimes - (2).

    c.   I struggle to make healthy choices - (3).

14. What's your comfort level with taking risks?

    a.   Low - (1).

    b.   Medium - (2).

    c.   High - (3).

15. Do you consider yourself:

    a.   Future orientated with big plans and clear goals - (1).

    b.   Informed by the past, hopeful about the future and aspiring to live in the moment - (2).

    c.   Present orientated, it's all about what feels good now - (3).

16. How would you characterize yourself as a student?

    a. Stellar - (1).

    b. Solid - (2).

    c. Slacker - (3).

17. When you first wake up in the morning are you:

    a. Bright eyed - (1).

    b. Dazed but not confused - (2).

    c. Groggy, eyelids made of cement - (3).

18. How would you describe your appetite within half an hour of waking?

    a. Very hungry - (1).

    b. Hungry - (2).

    c. Not at all hungry - (3).

19. How often do you suffer from insomnia symptoms?

    a. Rarely, only when adjusting to a new time zone - (1).

    b. Occasionally, when going through a rough time or are stressed out - (2).

    c. Chronically, it comes in waves - (3).

20. How would you describe your overall life satisfaction?

    a. High - (1).

    b. Good - (2).

    c. Low - (3).

Your Results - Are You a Lion, Bear or Wolf?

Go back over all your answers from 11 to 30, then total up the points allocated to each answer.

This will then give you a total score, then using the below scoring system you can then determine which chronotype you are from the below options:

Lion: 19 - 32.

Bear: 33 -47.

Wolf: 48 - 61.

Lion, Bear, Wolf or Dolphin?

Are You a Lion?

Most alert: Noon.

Most productive: Morning.

Naps: Almost never.

- Conscientious.
- Stable.
- Practical.
- Optimistic.
- Overachieving.
- Focused and prioritises health.
- Seeks positive interaction.
- Strategising.

Are You a Bear?

Most alert: Mid-morning to early afternoon.

Most productive: Late morning.

Naps: Weekends on the sofa.

- Cautious.
- Extroverted.
- Friendly.
- Open minded.
- Easy to talk to.
- Avoids conflict.

- Aspires to be healthy.
- Prioritises happiness.
- Takes comfort in the familiar.

Are You a Wolf?

Most alert: 7pm.

Most productive: Late morning and late evening.

Naps: Tempting, however if a wolf sleeps in the day, they won't sleep at night, so not worth it.

- Impulsive.
- Pessimistic.
- Creative.
- Moody.
- A risk-taker.
- Prioritises pleasure.
- Reacts with emotional intensity.

Are You a Dolphin?

Most alert: Late at night.

Most productive: Spurts throughout the day.

Naps: They try to nap to catch up on sleep however can't quite make it happen.

- Cautious
- Introverted.
- Neurotic.
- Intelligent.
- Avoids risky situations.

- Strives for perfection.
- Obsessive compulsive tendencies.
- Fixated on details.

"Without enough sleep, we all become tall two-year-olds."

— JoJo Jensen

REMOVE...
LET'S JUST SAY I WON'T MISS YOU!

TURN IT OFF, SO YOU TURN OFF 6

Where Did it All Go So Wrong?

And yes, it did, so badly!

I have noticed in my mere four decades on this planet that a lot of things that are supposed to be helping us, tech in particular, though in theory amazing, the harsh reality is that it actually makes us less efficient.

Technology and sleep are no different.

Years ago, when we left the office, pretty much all our work stuff stayed in the office, except perhaps for a few papers. Never mind the fact that those papers didn't radiate out bright blue light late into the night, tricking our bodies into thinking it's morning sunlight and reducing our melatonin levels by up to 25%.

Your Favourite Sleep Hormone

Melatonin, also known as the "Sleep Hormone", is critical to our sleep every night as it slows the body down, ready for a great night's sleep.

My objective for you with this chapter, is to make everything as simple as possible to action which is why I focus on the "hows" and not the "whys".

All light suppresses melatonin. However, some lights are worse than others. The flip of this is that low light boosts melatonin, which is exactly what we want!

Devices that produce dangerous levels of short-wave blue light, both the obvious and not so obvious:

- TVs.
- Computers.
- Mobile phones & tablets.
- Bright blue lights on alarm clocks, plus other electronics in the bedroom.
- LED Spotlights.

Where Things Get Really Simple

So, to ensure you boost your melatonin at night, there are a few super simple things to do:

1. Get natural sunlight as early as possible in the day. Yes, that means you have to leave the house in the morning! Anytime is better than none. However, the sunlight gained first thing will boost melatonin production more than sunlight later in the day.

2. From around 7pm (I appreciate in summer it's still light), start to dim your lights. If you don't have dimmer switches, get them, or if you can't be bothered to do this - which I get, as it's another thing to do - or if it's out of your budget, have fewer lights on.

3. If you have bright white LED spotlights, it's a good idea to stop using them after 7pm as these are a massive bolt of intense blue light zapped right into your eyes, just at the time when that's the last thing you need.

A good way is to keep hall or landing lights on, providing ambient light to the rooms you're in by keeping the doors open while not being blasted directly from light fittings in the room where you are.

4. Turn off all electrical devices an hour before bedtime, yes that includes the TV! This is a lot easier than it may sound, as if you create an evening "Sleep Routine", by the time you've showered, locked up, read the kids stories, got clothes ready for work tomorrow, read before bed etc, this will amount to around an hour. Easy!

5. The other tiny yet highly effective change is using your phone's blue light filter on an Android or Night Shift mode on iOS.

6. Finally, one habit I do religiously for weeks, then forget all about (annoyingly!) is blue light blocker glasses. These are great. I do notice an improvement in my sleep when using them.

Your Sleep Checklist - Time for You to Turn it OFF

1. Are you on electrical devices like phones tablets and laptops in bed or towards the end of the evening, if so, what time is their use stopped?

2. Do you have a TV in your bedroom and is it used?

3. Do you have bright spotlights throughout the house?

4. Do you use your phone and PC/laptop's blue light filter?

Your Action Plan – STOP!! Waking Up Tired.

1. Get natural sunlight as early as possible in the day.

2. From around 7pm, start to dim your household lights.

3. Turn off all electrical devices an hour before bedtime (whenever this is for you).

4. Turn on your phone's blue light filter NOW. It will take you 30 seconds.

5. Wear blue light blocker glasses from 2pm if in an office or from 5pm at home.

Always remember keep things simple and start small! Pick just one thing to action this week, then forget the rest until you have made that one action point a habit. Rinse, repeat...

Your Personal Sleep Notes

"The nicest thing for me is sleep,
then at least I can dream."

-Marilyn Monroe

THEY'RE A PAIN IN THE NECK 7

Though I write about sleep and have spent the last twenty years of my life optimising my sleep and coaching others on the holy grail of health and longevity, I didn't cover this critical sleep lesson for a long time, and yet it's so important!

It came to a head one night, just before I was to record all the training material for my Sleep Mastery Coaching Program. I'd spent the previous few months designing and writing the course before finally putting all the downloads together, and on this particular night I found myself in the most excruciating pain.

Conversely, I was pleased that it happened (although not at the time) as I was then able to gather even greater insights into the mechanism of optimum sleep and add it to the course before recording it.

So, what had happened? Earlier that day I was stretching my neck and pushed it to its limits. Well, judging by the pain I was in, in fact way beyond my limits

The fun didn't stop there either, as every time I moved, even slightly throughout the night, the type of movements that would typically go unnoticed, I awoke each time in intense pain.

The Power of a Bad Back

This reminded me of a client I had on this matter, I'd not previously thought about this angle from a proactive perspective. It was always more from a reactive perspective when a client had an issue.

This particular client was experiencing the most intense back pain, which was so great that he could not sleep for weeks on end, and I mean weeks!

Upon hearing this, I knew straight away that his years of rugby, bad posture and never having had a massage in his entire life, combined with not bothering to stretch for the last decade, were the root causes of his problems and, in turn, sleepless nights.

So I recommended him to a local sports masseuse. Then a few days later, after just two massages, unbelievable for him (though very obvious to me) he was able to sleep a lot better.

The ultimate source of his sleepless nights was his bad posture, sedentary lifestyle and lack of stretching. Not a lack of massages, as this was simply the tonic to his bad habits. It was the massages that REMOVED the pain. However, without improvements in his posture, a regular stretching regime and a continued sedentary lifestyle, in a few weeks or months his pain would simply return.

Now, I appreciate a massage won't remove the pain for everyone, and may be out of budget for some, however, it serves as a great example of how something as every day as pain can completely devastate your sleep, mood, energy and ultimately happiness and enjoyment from life.

I personally have two massages a week, so it wasn't long before my next massage to rectify this issue, combined with the simple fact that time is a great healer. This allowed my severe pain to return to normal levels in a matter of days. Or another option could be, asking a partner or friend to do this for you. You will be amazed by the difference even this makes.

Remove the Source of Your Pain, Don't Mask the Pain

If you have pain, or more likely for most, you find yourself in any pain in the future, don't take this lying down (pun intended!).

Find out what's causing the problem, then don't try to MASK the pain, e.g. alcohol and painkillers. Ensure you FIX the pain by finding the root cause. In the example above, my client had a considerable number of tight muscles that had not been stretched or massaged for decades, having endured years of rugby and bad posture, the latter two being the ultimate source of his problems.

Many different sources of pain can keep people up during the night. It's your job to become aware of this, then make the direct link between this and what is causing your sleep problems, and finally, take action with a health practitioner to FIX (not mask) the problem.

Sleeping Position

Sleeping position can considerably reduce any pain you currently have, while you are in the process of getting it fixed and can be itself a source of pain. I cover sleep positions in a lot more detail in a later chapter. However, it's worth noting now, as I want you to be aware of this aspect and not have to endure another few weeks of pain before this issue is resolved. So, try different positions.

Your main options for improvements are:

1. Back sleeping.
2. Side sleeping.

Another really handy tip that can make sleeping on your side so much comfier is using a pillow between your legs. Yes, you heard that right, and it really does work!

Those With Multiple Sclerosis

Another client of mine, James, who has MS, would often have a terrible night's sleep, unsurprisingly. However, we decided to focus on a FIX for him and NOT a mask.

We broke down his daily habits to find out what was triggering his inflammation, and before long, we could see that he had a lot of highly inflammatory based habits, which would have most likely caused the MS in the first place.

So, we changed a few things for him, and we always start slowly to make it easy to action. This then allows us to see results quickly and in turn, increase the uptake of further significant actions.

There was nothing significant to change. He would reduce his nightly alcohol drinking from five drinks to three drinks, have a cold shower at some point during the day, take a tablespoon of turmeric daily, 1,000mg of vitamin C daily and increase his water intake (filtered, of course!).

I also from time to time let him use my Hyperbaric Oxygen Chamber and his sleep went through the roof!

Daily Painful Things to Be Aware of…

A lot of these I appreciate is common sense. However, simply by making you aware of the considerable impact these have on your sleep, you will now (hopefully) think twice about them, as you are pre-warned and aware of these dangers.

Sunburn

This is a simple one. Just be aware of the sun's intensity when out and about with little (or perhaps no) clothes on. Where in the world you are, the time of year it is and the time of day, are the key factors to pay attention to.

Aim to stay in the shade as much as possible, wear cool yet protective clothing, and use high-quality "natural" sun lotions to protect against intense sunlight. Though this is not the time or place to address this, I do have doubts about a lot of the chemicals used in mainstream sun protection.

That said, always remember that the sun is good for you, just not excessive sun.

When you have tight sun burnt skin, good luck with sleeping! Never mind the intense heat radiating from you, the scabbed or broken sunburnt skin makes for several unpleasant nights and equally harder to heal days.

When hot, ask yourself how long I can stay in this before it wrecks my sleep tonight.

Bites & Rashes.

All these everyday irritants work along the same lines, waking you up and keeping you awake while trying to sleep.

If you live somewhere that has a problem with mosquitoes, for example, first things first would be to keep windows closed to limit the number of biting insects in your bedroom at night.

Look to sleep inside a net if there is no way of stopping the pesky intruders from entering your bedroom. In some countries, the number of flying irritants is just too overwhelming, and this is your safest bet.

A great and surprising trick I have learnt is that by having a fan in your bedroom directed at you, the pesky insects find it very difficult to fly over you. This is due to the air turbulence, as I used to get bit loads until I found this great game changer by accident.

And if they can't get to you, it means they can't bite you! That simple. Also don't forget quinine i.e. tonic water, just without the gin, is also amazing for this. Just ask British army officers in India 100 years ago! While another natural source is lavender.

So, you are now spoiled for choice when it comes to avoiding getting bit - fans, nets, tonic water and lavender!

Intense Exercise

If you have ever lifted weights or moved anything heavy or unusual to what your body typically does, you will know this one all too well!

Yes, I know you are keen to get big muscles to impress the love interest in your life in super-quick time. However, the price you pay is having excruciatingly sore muscles for days on end.

These painful muscles, aside from being highly annoying for a few days, will, if pushed hard enough, also keep you up at night. In turn, rather detrimental to you as without a good sleep you won't be able to perform at your best in the gym, never mind having the charm and quick wit to impress those hotties into making their clothes look far better on your bedroom floor, than on them!

The key is to progress consistently and not to the point that you will be in agony for days.

Some instances, like emergencies where you have to lift randomly shaped heavy objects in funny angles, can't be helped, but for most things it can.

Stay alert to such situations for the sake of tomorrow!

Banging Hard Objects

This will affect more women than men, as more women associate themselves as being clumsy than men (not the banging hard objects!).

First off, you aren't clumsy. You just think you are. This makes you believe you are clumsy, and the mind then creates situations to back up your false beliefs.

I appreciate some people may have genetic or ill health issues that will make this happen more, though generally this is a mindset thing.

Simply being consciously aware of your environment and any aspects that could be problematic will significantly reduce the number of hard objects banged!

However, the big one is stop rushing. When you rush, mistakes happen. Stay calm, relaxed and, in turn, controlled. This will result in far fewer bumps and bruises.

To save a few seconds or even minutes rushing, it's just simply not worth the many sleepless nights from the pain a knock to the body or head will bring!

Plus, there are many more ways that by exposing yourself to unnecessary problems you can be playing havoc on your sleep and energy levels the next day. These are just the ones that I have experienced in my sleep journey.

Chronic Pain

I appreciate I haven't covered chronic pain; however, I strongly recommend if this is an issue for you, that you read my first book in the STOP!! Series. STOP!! Killing Yourself...The Beginners Guide to Living Longer.

A lot of issues for those with chronic pain are inflammation based and this book gives great detail on easy yet very effective ways to reduce your inflammation. It might not cure you, but it will make life for you a lot easier - never mind you'll get better sleep!

Your Sleep Checklist - Stop the Pain in the Neck

1. Do you have a bad neck, back, arm, leg or any other pain that keeps you up at night?

_____

_____

_____

2. Do you know the source of this pain and why you have it?

_____

_____

_____

3. Do you have regular massages?

_____

_____

_____

4. Do you wake up with pains that you didn't have the night before often?

_____

_____

_____

Your Action Plan – STOP!! Waking Up Tired.

1. Ask yourself, do you have any pains that keep you up at night?

2. Spend some time understanding what this pain is. Dr Google is always there for you, and they may even provide you with some guidance!

3. Consider having regular sports massages and visiting an osteopath or a physiotherapist. Remember you want to fix the cause, not simply alleviate the pain. Which may mean simply changing your posture at your desk or when you walk and other lifestyle habits.

4. Visit a healthcare practitioner to get it FIXED. Avoid painkillers except in extreme cases as they wreck your gut biome.

5. Pay attention to your environment, whether this is sun intensity, insects and animals, exercising too hard or general clumsiness.

Your Personal Sleep Notes

"The best bridge between despair and hope is a good night's sleep."

— E. Joseph Cossman

STOP PISSING ABOUT AT NIGHT   8

Would you like to stop pissing at night?

Late night pissing is one of those very annoying nightly activities that for men, as the years go by, increase in frequency (and annoyance).

Yet so simple to fix.

For those of you reading this, you are most likely very aware of returning to bed and then simply lying there awake for hours, unable to get back to sleep, tossing and turning.

However, the main reason why it's such a big problem, is lurking behind the surface.

First off, if you are lucky enough that when you get back into bed, you then go straight back to sleep, and for some of you, you are now probably thinking to yourself in a smug fashion, yep that's me alright!

Well think again! As you have now already broken your sleep cycle and will have most likely awoken yourself up from the holy grail of sleep, "Deep Sleep".

Once you have broken this, best case, you have now significantly reduced the amount of deep sleep you get that night. However, for most of you, that is it folks! Your deep sleep for this night is now over and you will now have to wait again until tomorrow night for your deep sleep fix! That is of course, if you don't pee again tomorrow night…

Then there are those who once they have left the bed and gone to the bathroom for that late night pee, they get back into bed and BOOM, they just lie there for hours, unable to sleep.

At least with this group, they know the damage late night pissing is doing to them and are therefore highly motivated, to make the changes we are going to discuss now.

The fun doesn't stop there either… As it gets even worse if you then decide to put the lights on in order to stop you stubbing your toe in the dark!

Better is to familiarise yourself with the walk to your loo and take it slowly, so not to wake yourself up with bright bathroom lights and being able to leave your lights OFF!

I am going to jump straight in and give you some of the simple yet highly effective ways I overcome the dreaded late night "piss stop".

Make Your Last 5pm

What I am about to tell you is so simple, yet it will transform not just your sleep but your entire life, by waking up a lot more energised than you presently are!

In fact, this one transformed British Lions rugby international, Gareth Cooper's sleep!

One of the easiest and most underrated sleep optimising tactics, is simply removing that late night drink! And I don't mean alcohol, I mean any liquid.

Most likely you are a male over forty reading this and if not, you soon will be! And for the women it's a good opportunity to understand what men go through with their bladders.

So, for the men, you will be fully aware that in the last few years you needing to go for a late-night pee has pretty much come out of nowhere, plus from speaking with older men than me, this aspect of needing a pee at night will only get worse.

Therefore, the easiest and simplest solution is to simply cut out liquids after 5pm!

Yes, at first this may be met with huge resistance and also a "no way" from you, it can't be that simple, can it?

Well, yes, it is, as I have tested this at forty. I am now forty-two writing this and any time I think I am above this law, well think again Ralphy boy, you aren't!

Take last Thursday for example, I had three pints with friends very unexpectedly, a last-minute thing as a friend cancelled our walk that evening annoyingly. So, I had just sat down to read for the evening and then he called saying he was now in a pub barely two minutes' walk from me, in fact I could even see them both from my window, so, as I had not seen him for some time, I decided to pop in and join them.

I left them at 9pm, was asleep for 9.30pm and yet there I was at around 2am pissing the night away!

If you don't believe me or how powerful this is, test it out for yourself. And I can guarantee the older you are, the more powerful the results will be for you! This is an absolute game changer.

Of course, if you are extremely thirsty, I am not saying after 5pm you have to die of thirst, far from it. I am saying just be very conscious of what liquids you drink after 5pm. The odd sips here and there are fine of course, I am meaning a full glass of liquid.

If this one is a bit tricky at first for you, start by not drinking any liquids for an hour before bed for the first week, then two hours before bed for the second week and finally for the third week, you are down to the magic four hours before bed, which is just where you want to be.

Slowly but surely, is nearly always the best way to implement new habits. For some of you the issue will be that bad that you will simply stop drinking liquids at 5pm and that's it done.

For others who don't think it's that bad an issue waking up at night for a pee, then you might start implementing this over a three week period as suggested above to see how it works for you.

Your Sleep Checklist – To Stop Pissing at Night

1. What time do you stop consuming liquids in the day?

2. Do you wake up in the night for a pee?

3. Do you wake up slightly before your alarm goes off as your bladder is full?

4. If you wake up in the night for a pee, can you then get back to sleep?

Your Action Plan – STOP!! Waking Up Tired.

1. Focus your liquid consumption in the mornings and early afternoons.

2. Look to stop consuming liquids from 5pm.

3. If you do need to drink after this time, be conscious of having the absolute bare minimum required to quench your thirst.

Your Personal Sleep Notes

"I'm so good at sleeping that I can do it with my eyes closed."

— Anonymous

MAKE YOUR LAST MIDDAY **9**

Welcome to Generation Stimulation

I t certainly DOESN'T, give you wings, that's for sure…

The very nature of a stimulant is to make you more alert and provide you with more energy, which is the exact opposite of what one needs come bedtime!

For this reason, by giving yourself many hours between stimulant consumption and bedtime, most of the effects from stimulants like caffeine and energy drinks will have diminished to low levels, though still in your system in small doses, now allowing you to sleep.

Think about it, do you want to be taking something that stimulates you at the very time you want to be approaching your sleep phase, therefore early evening? Never mind, late evening!

For those of you who are reliant on stimulants, you will absolutely love the big, quick wins you are about to get, not just for your sleep, but your life as a whole.

Energy Drinks

There are huge overlaps with the stimulating effect of coffee, so I'll keep things simple and group coffee and energy drinks in the same category.

Plus, I will introduce you briefly to their dangerous sugar levels. A can of the Monster energy drink has 55 grams of sugar! This is absolute and utter pure living hell for your body. This is two to five times my daily sugar in one drink!

Make midday your last and, if you really have to, 2pm at the very latest.

Make Your Last Midday

This may scare some of you…

Coffee ideally needs to be stopped at midday. What? I hear you all say: "no way Ralph! Piss off…"

Well, if you are going to get the most benefits out of your life, it's a good habit to form and one I adhere to pretty much every day.

However, if you want to keep having a rubbish sleep and waking up tired, then just ignore this and carry on with your destructive habits, as it isn't my sleep being affected!

Though annoyingly, my satisfaction from coaching you will be affected, as I get great joy from seeing the massive improvements, I make to people's lives…Buy hey, perhaps just not yours!

OK, so here's the deal: if you can't bring yourself to do the midday day cut-off thing, 2pm is a great starting point for you! Let me explain how I have fully optimised this for myself.

I have two cups of organic mycotoxin coffee, freshly ground, daily, except for Sundays. Why Sundays? I like to give my body a caffeine break. Plus most months, I will also go a week without coffee to stop my body from getting used to its effects.

I have my first cup of coffee around 7am. I wake up at 5.30am every morning and deliberately give myself at least an hour before my first cup of coffee, though the longer the better, which is why it's generally around one to two hours from waking.

I do this because I want to benefit from the natural rise in my cortisol levels when I first wake, as coffee also boosts my cortisol levels. However, I like the coffee boost benefits to kick in when my natural cortisol levels start to drop.

Brief side point: cortisol is an essential hormone; without it we would die and indeed it is not the monster it is made out to be. Though if you are constantly stressed, it becomes perilous. That's the critical importance between acute and chronic inflammation.

Then my final cup of coffee is around 10am. I have two cups daily, as two to three cups have been proven to be the best for longevity and general wellbeing.

This will really bring you significant changes in your sleep and, therefore, your life. As we all know, sleeping better means a better life in every aspect, from mood, energy, emotions, productivity and happiness.

Coffee Shops

A few areas where I can get tempted and even succumb, even though this is the very blueprint that I live by "most days", it's not something I do every single day, just "most" days.

So, if I have a meeting in a coffee shop, then yes, at 3pm I will have a coffee, and if it's a Saturday, I have even been known to have a coffee up to 4pm.

Drinking Alcohol

I have had an interesting and complicated relationship with alcohol over the years, which was the main motivation for my first book on living longer, as I was conscious of the disruption it has played on my sleep over the years. It was for this reason I was so focused on improving my sleep, as I realised this was a key to offsetting the very obvious effects that alcohol has had on my life after excessive partying.

I don't want to delve too deeply into alcohol, as it's a very emotional topic for a lot of people. Plus, there are other experts better suited for anyone who has a problem with this poisonous substance, and yes, I do take alcohol from time to time on special occasions, such as holidays, sunny days, birthdays and Christmas, though in an ideal world, it would be just twice a year, on my birthday, with my best friend and at Christmas with my sister.

In a nutshell, which you already know, and this is simply a reminder, it really fucks with your sleep. It will affect the big ones, namely your REM. That's it. I can't gloss over it any other way.

In a nutshell, which you already know, and this is simply a reminder; alcohol really fucks with your sleep. It will affect the big ones, namely your REM. That's it. I can't gloss over it any other way.

Never mind if you are a bloke and drink pints, then it's going to see you visiting the loo around one visit per two pints consumed after the age of forty. Then for those over sixty, it may even be one loo visit per pint, lucky you!

There we go, that's it. I kept this short and sweet as I know no one wants to be lectured about their drinking, as they have a husband or wife for that!

Your Sleep Checklist - Make Your Last Midday

1. What time is your last coffee of the day?

2. Do you drink alcohol most evenings?

3. Do you drink energy drinks and if so, how many and what time is your last?

4. Do you take any other types of stimulants?

Your Action Plan – STOP!! Waking Up Tired.

1. Focus your stimulant consumption in your mornings.

2. Make midday your last, with 2pm being the hard cut-off, while getting used to this.

3. See energy drinks for what they are - hazardous liquids, full of poison, sorry, I mean sugar. If you want the energy boost, switch to coffee.

Your Personal Sleep Notes

"A well-spent day brings happy sleep."

— Leonardo da Vinci

ONE OF THE BEST WAYS TO WAKE UP OBESE AND TIRED!

10

Pay Attention to The Time you Eat

This is one of the big ones! And I mean, one of the BIG ones.

So, let's get straight to the point. Late night eating directs a large amount of your blood to your stomach, which in turn takes blood away from the rest of your body, where it is needed to repair, restore and cleanse your body of the daily stresses it endures, when you are asleep.

By eating within four hours of sleep, you are depriving your body of this amazing bodily function, one that optimises you, ready for the next day.

Though I am sure the exact amount of time varies between individuals, I have tested that two hours, is simply not enough, when it comes to that last mouthful and the time between your head hitting that pillow of yours!

Three hours is the absolute minimum, and I mean the absolute minimum, from your last meal to bedtime.

Personally, I make it four hours being my typical daily habit, i.e. my last meal is 5pm and lights out 9.30pm.

Plus, while we are on the subject of mealtimes, keeping them consistent, is also great for your circadian rhythm AND don't forget food consumed late at night is more likely to be stored as fat than used as energy!

In fact, for those of you reluctant to do this one, just think how much more weight you will gain, if you keep eating late at night!

Eating Out & Socialising

I know what you're now thinking and going to say next, but Ralph, what about business meals and socialising with friends over dinner on the weekends?

This one, I appreciate is not quite as easy as day-to-day home life. However, let me explain what I have done to protect myself from the dangers of late-night eating.

First off, if someone wants a business dinner; I suggest you make this a late lunch. Easy, as this now bats off most issues here when it comes to late night eating.

Secondly, if that's not ideal for them, I suggest going for dinner at 5pm, which they will then often counter with 7pm from the originally suggested 8pm. I will then say, well I could be forced to do 6pm but that's my absolute latest, as I really can't eat after that, as it makes me really tired the next day and effects my work performance.

This is the key thing to say, as by planting the seed as to what it does to you they will often, though not always, think oh shit, could it be doing the same to me and my sleep? Sometimes, they may ask why eating late will affect their sleep? Which is when you explain why, selling them on the benefits as well.

If it's dinner with just one friend, as all my friends now know my stance on this, and of course they know I am a sleep, stress and longevity coach, so, they listen to my advice and in fact a few now have stopped going out for dinner late at night themselves, independently of me.

That one for me is easy, however when you have a one-on-one interaction with someone you know well, it's an easy sell as your friends will mainly want what's best for you and understand your reasons.

The hard one though, is big groups of friends and strangers, even more so on a Friday or Saturday night. Even if you are organising this evening, getting the buy in from 10 to 20 people to eat at 6pm, is only likely to mean some people won't accept the invitation.

You have two options here:

1. If dinner would normally be 8pm or even 9pm, bring this slightly forward to 7pm, most people won't have a big enough issue with that time to stop them attending, even if they would like it to be later. I appreciate you now won't finish eating until 8pm-ish, though if you are out for dinner, you are certainly going to be going to bed later than normal anyway, most likely around 11pm to 12pm, which gives you three to four hours between eating and sleeping.

2. Your second option if things are later than this and you have no control over the event and still want to attend, is to simply have your main meal around 5pm as normal, then at the dinner, simply order a starter for your main, or as I have been known to do, a child's meal. Yes, you should see people's faces when I order it!

This really is one of those lifestyle changes that you want to start slowly and in super small steps. Otherwise it will be too big a shock to you and your family's already hardwired habits.

I would suggest if you are eating at 8pm currently, then perhaps experiment with 7.30pm for a few weeks, which is such an easy transition and no one will even notice. Then once accustomed to that, bring it forward to 7pm, again for another few weeks.

For those of you going to bed at around 11pm, this is a very suitable time and not much of an issue over a few weeks or months to transition. However, for those sleeping a bit earlier at around 10pm, I would really recommend bringing that forward to 6.30pm or in an ideal world 6pm. I don't eat after 6pm with my last supper typically around 5pm, though I go to sleep at 9.30pm. Perhaps this is why I am currently single!

Your Sleep Checklist - Stop Eating Late at Night

1. **What time do you eat you last meal of the day?**

2. **Do you snack or consume any additional food later in the evening?**

3. **Do you feel full or bloated when you go to bed?**

4. **Do you wake up still full from the night before?**

Your Action Plan – STOP!! Waking Up Tired.

1. Make your last meal of the day, the last thing you eat for the day i.e. no snacks after your dinner or supper.

2. Aim to finish your last meal of the day four hours before bedtime i.e. if you sleep at 10pm, aim to start eating at 5.30pm, so that you are all finished by 6pm, giving you a clear four hours between eating and sleep.

Your Personal Sleep Notes

"Man is a genius when he is dreaming."

— Akira Kurosawa, Japanese Film Director

WHAT YOU EAT EFFECTS YOUR SLEEP

11

I t's not just the time you eat however, as certain foods eaten in the evening will play havoc with your sleep.

It is for this reason I have dedicated an entire chapter on the worst offenders for you and how they prevent a great night's sleep.

These are in no particular order as they are all pretty potent:

1. Cheese and dairy
2. Dark chocolate.
3. Tomatoes & Onions.
4. Curry.
5. Ice Cream & Sugary Friends.
6. Crisps.
7. Fatty Processed Food.

Cheese and dairy

Though I did say there was no order, this has to be number one and number one for a reason.

Cheese is rather bad at night due to the high levels of an amino acid called tyramine that makes us feel alert and awake. It activates your adrenal glands to release adrenaline. The effects can last for a few hours which is not so good at night!

As with everything I teach, I do the research and then run the tests, and cheese was no different. So last Sunday, to put this to the test, I ate a thick slice of organic mature cheddar, not a massive amount by any means.

Then when I tested my deep sleep for that evening, it came in at a very costly experiment, having just gotten 23 minutes of deep sleep Now put that into context, as I typically get between two and one-and-a-half hours of deep sleep, you can see how destructive this.

This sadly means no pizza while watching a late-night film, very annoying!

Dark Chocolate

I learnt this one the hard way, having not realised the time and eating some at 4pm, I eat a lot of 85% dark chocolate as it's better for you.

Dark chocolate contains caffeine and like we have just covered on the coffee front, for the same reasons this one needs to be kept to a morning and early afternoon snack.

Tomatoes & Onions

These two are on the list due to their ability to cause heartburn or acid reflux, I tend not to eat these in general except for my beloved pizza, of course!

In a nutshell, once you are horizontal in bed, you lose the beneficial gravitational pull stopping the acidity in the tomatoes consumed from rising from your oesophagus and keeping them very much where they need to be, in your stomach.

For similar reasons, onions also create gas and again, when lying down, you limit the effects of gravity for keeping this unwanted gas where it needs to stay.

Curry

It pains me to write this as I have a weekly curry! And as I write I am quite literally salivating over the thought of having a curry and even thinking of stopping for the day, going to my local curry house, yet it's only 3pm, and I've just eaten!

However, much to my friend Laptop Tom (he takes his laptop everywhere with him and I mean everywhere, of which I like to tease him over, hence his nickname!) original despair, we have now gotten into a habit on a Friday or Saturday of eating our weekly meal out now at 5.30pm. In fact, he is now even a convert!

Though saying that, I have a korma which has minimal spices. For those who prefer the spicier things in life, there are a few things you need to know.

The spices in curries and anything else with a kick, like mustard, contain high levels of a chemical called capsaicin.

It's this capsaicin that interferes with your body's temperature regulating system and raises your temperature. This is why you feel hot after eating something spicy!

And what is the one thing your body likes to be when it sleeps? Yes, you've guessed it, cool. So, eating something that makes you hot will make sleep difficult for you.

This is before we even cover that to digest such spices, we will need a lot more energy than for other food!

Ice Cream

Ok so pizza and curry are now off limits late at night, but no way to ice cream as well, Ralph? What are we going to do on a Saturday film night?

I know it's painful, but it's no different for me, either! As pizza, curry and ice cream are my favourites.

In fact, as a brief side note, it took me over two years to not always have ice cream in the house. It started off initially, to every other week, then once a month, to then a few times a year which is where I am now. Not easy, but certainly easier now…

We all know ice cream is full of sugar, this is nothing new. However, did you know that sugar plays absolute havoc with your sleep?

When you stop to think about it, it's actually quite obvious, as again, we all know about sugar spikes, which of course, ice cream, doughnuts, fruit juices etc are all going to cause. However, this is the bit you perhaps haven't thought of, is that what goes up, must come down…

And guess what happens when you come down? Your adrenal glands are alerted to this emergency. Resulting in increased cortisol levels, which is great for when we wake up first thing in the morning, giving us, quite literally, our get up and go. However not so good when we want to relax and sleep.

Obviously, if you are eating this sugar late at night, the crash will then of course occur when you are or were asleep! Which may even wake you up and at least will break any deep sleep you were experiencing.

Crisps

These are salty buggers! And it's this salt fest that causes your body to dehydrate, increasing your water retention levels and increasing your tiredness the next day.

High levels of salt contribute to highly disrupted sleep, or simply put, stop you from getting the high-quality holy grail of deep sleep, though ironically increases your REM, giving you nightmares.

After high levels of salt, it now takes longer to fall asleep while also providing you with highly disruptive deep sleep.

The fun doesn't stop there either, as they are not only salty but also greasy, which can impact your sweet dreams and turn them into nightmares! Think double whammy here - salt and grease.

This also ignores the fact they are full of pesticides, herbicides, etc., oxidised vegetable oils, and are highly processed. While adding no nutritional value. However, this is not a nutritional book, this is a sleep book, so we will stop there!

High Fat Foods

I appreciate there is going to be a lot of overlap here. However, high fat foods such as ice cream come under other categories, just like burgers, which are also full of grease and highly processed.

Fatty foods take longer to digest, as they are harder to digest. This means while you are asleep your body is flat out, pun intended, working hard to digest this high fat food.

Your Sleep Checklist - What You Eat

1. Do you eat cheese, tomatoes, onions, curry, or processed foods after 6pm?

    _____

    _____

    _____

2. Do you eat chocolate, ice cream, sugary foods and crisps after 6pm?

    _____

    _____

    _____

Your Action Plan – STOP!! Waking Up Tired.

1. Avoid spicy foods after 6pm.

2. Avoid cheese after 6pm.

3. Avoid sugar after 6pm.

4. Avoid fatty foods after 6pm.

Your Personal Sleep Notes

"We are such stuff as dreams are made on."

— William Shakespeare

ARE YOUR MEDS GIVING YOU NIGHTMARES?

A s people get older, they seem to acquire more money, larger waistlines and more health conditions…

Sadly, with health conditions, rather than fixing the root cause of the problem, people often go for the easy option, the quick fix, and the doctors certainly facilitate you in that easy option.

Opting for quick-fix medications to mask your underlying health issues, you may find yourself prescribed to medicines that you think are good for you, but are actually causing you more harm than good.

I am no pharmacist or doctor, so **please speak with your health care provider** before making any changes; however, I will outline very popular medications that you may be taking that are known to interfere with great sleep.

In light of this, I have put together the top seven forms of medication that could be disrupting your sleep. A few types of medication that I haven't covered due to the chapter getting way too long are ACE Inhibitors, ARBs and Glucosamine.

The Top 7 Medications That Cause Insomnia

1. Statins.
2. Beta-blockers.
3. Alpha-blockers.
4. Antidepressants.
5. Cholinesterase inhibitors.
6. Corticosteroids.
7. Antihistamines.

Statins

A very popular prescription drug used to treat those with high cholesterol. They cause insomnia and sleep interruption due to their most common side effect of muscle pain, which can keep you up at night.

Types of statins include:

1. Lovastatin.
2. Atorvastatin.
3. Rosuvastatin.
4. Simvastatin.

Typical brand names include:

1. Mevacor.
2. Lipitor.
3. Crestor.
4. Zocor.

By far the most common complaint related to sleep from statins involves muscle pain. These can keep those on statins up at night, the duration varies from person to person, and therefore, the resultant impact on one's sleep varies.

The worst offenders seem to be Mevacor, Lipitor, Zocor and Vytorin. These are all fat-soluble statins. These statins affect your sleep more because they can penetrate cell membranes easier, penetrating the blood/brain barrier, which protects your brain from unwelcome chemicals in the blood.

Speak with your doctor about healthy lifestyle alternatives for those who are taking these from a prevention perspective i.e. slightly higher cholesterol levels as opposed actually to having heart disease.

Ironically, one of the best things for your health is… sleep! Go figure…

Beta Blockers

They are typically prescribed for those with high blood pressure (hypertension) and abnormal heartbeats (arrhythmias).

Beta bockers lower your blood pressure and slow your heart rate by blocking your adrenaline hormone. Beta-blockers are also used to treat tremors, migraines and angina.

Types of beta blockers include:

1. Timolol.
2. Sotalol.
3. Propranolol.
4. Metoprolol.
5. Carvedilol.
6. Atenolol.

Typical brand names include:

1. Timoptic.
2. Betapace.
3. Inderal.

4. Lopressor.
5. Coreg.
6. Tenormin.

The best bit about beta blockers is that they give you nightmares! Thank you doctor…

Don't think the fun stops there either, as they are well known for waking up users by inhibiting the night time secretion of one of our most important hormones for great health, melatonin. I can't stress enough how important this hormone is to a long and happy life.

Alpha Blockers

These are typically prescribed for various health conditions, with high blood pressure and Raynaud's disease being the most popular use for them.

They help keep small blood vessels open and relax muscles. Alpha-blockers do this by reducing the effects of the hormone norepinephrine (also called noradrenaline), which tightens the muscles in the walls of smaller arteries and veins. In turn, improves blood flow and lowers your blood pressure.

They are also sometimes used to help with urine flow for men with an enlarged prostate for the same reasons as relaxing muscles.

Types of alpha blockers include:

1. Alfuzosin.
2. Doxazosin.
3. Prazosin.
4. Silodosin.
5. Terazosin.
6. Tamsulosin.

Typical brand names include:

1. Uroxatral.
2. Cardura.
3. Minipress.
4. Rapaflo.
5. Hytrin.
6. Flomax.

Alpha-blockers decrease your REM (when you dream), a fundamental part of your daily sleep requirements. REM and deep sleep drop with age as it is, so you certainly don't need anything helping to worsen this key aspect of life.

Antidepressants

Or SSRIs, selective serotonin reuptake inhibitors. These are prescribed to those with mild forms of depression.

Antidepressants block the reabsorption of serotonin, a neurotransmitter in the brain. Blocking the reabsorption of serotonin makes more available to the brain.

As a side note, I personally take 5 HTP, a protein that naturally helps boost my serotonin to enhance my mood and help boost my sleep, plus serotonin is required to produce melatonin, the most essential hormone for sleep.

Types of antidepressants include:

1. Fluoxetine.
2. Sertraline.
3. Citalopram.
4. Escitalopram.
5. Fluvoxamine.
6. Paroxetine.

Typical brand names include:

1. Prozac.
2. Sarafem.
3. Zoloft.
4. Celexa.
5. Lexapro.
6. Luvox.
7. Paxil.

We don't quite know how antidepressants work, which makes this tough to answer why it affects sleep; however, the facts show it does. We just don't know how.

Sleep issues stem from mild tremors and agitation, with some people reporting insomnia. Again, super ironic is the very thing critical for depression, and, generally feeling great, is sleep.

Yet the things prescribed to help depression is stopping the very best thing to help with it. Again, go figure…

Cholinesterase Inhibitors

These are prescribed to treat those with forms of memory loss and mental changes for those individuals suffering from forms of dementia.

Types of cholinesterase inhibitors include:

1. Rivastigmine.
2. Galantamine.
3. Donepezil.

Typical brand names include:

1. Exelon.
2. Razadyne.
3. Aricept.

Aside from helping you feel sick and making you run to the bathroom to avoid soiling your underwear with diarrhoea, they, of course, play havoc with your sleep. Other side effects include muscle spasms and cramps, which will keep you up at night.

By blocking the breakdown of acetylcholine, you interfere with a neurotransmitter that is everywhere in the body and, surprisingly, not just in the brain by being a neurotransmitter.

Acetylcholine is critical for your memory, thought, alertness and judgement. The theory of how these drug works is by inhibiting the enzyme that breaks acetylcholine down you boost the amount available to the brain.

Corticosteroids

These have a wide range of uses, however, the common denominator is to treat forms of inflammation, so they are used to treat arthritis, gout and lupus.

Types of corticosteroids include:

1. Triamcinolone.
2. Prednisone.
3. Methylprednisolone.
4. Cortisone.

Typical brand names include:

1. Deltasone.
2. Sterapred.
3. Medrol.

Corticosteroids play havoc with your adrenal glands, which, as we all know, are responsible for managing your flight or fight response. Too much stress will keep you alert and unable to relax and sleep at night. Other side effects would include nightmares if you thought its side effects weren't bad enough already!

Antihistamines

Typically these are prescribed to help with allergic reactions and are also called nonsedating H1 antagonists. Original antihistamines would cause intense drowsiness due to their powerful suppression effects on the central nervous system.

They work by inhibiting the body's production of histamine. A chemical released when you have an allergic reaction to something. Hay fever is an excellent example with the resultant symptoms including running nose, watery eyes, blocked nose, sneezing and itching.

Types of antihistamines include:

1. Azelastine.
2. Cetirizine.
3. Desloratadine.
4. Fexofenadine.
5. Levocetirizine.
6. Loratadine.

Typical brand names include:

1. Astelin.
2. Zyrtec.
3. Clarinex.
4. Allegra.
5. Xyzal.
6. Claritin.

We have already covered one type of drug that blocks acetylcholine, cholinesterase inhibitors. You can expect a similar experience with antihistamines. However, as they typically only last for around eight hours within your body, simply taking them in the morning can quickly resolve their sleep-destroying properties.

Your Sleep Checklist – Medications

1. Are you on medication, if so, which kind?

2. If so, have you noticed a difference in your sleep since taking?

3. Have you looked for alternative natural remedies or medications?

4. Have you thought about improving your overall general health to gradually come off the medications?

Speak With Your Pharmacist or Doctor...

Ultimately this chapter is to give you an awareness that your main sleep issues can, in fact, be attributed to the medications you are taking.

Of course, for a lot of you who are not taking any medications, then this is not relevant; and, as with all medication, the side effects may not happen to you, but do take the time to evaluate whether you've become more tired or had less sleep since taking them. Then of course you need to weigh up the benefits long term to your health. I would recommend one of the first ports of call would be to establish with your doctor if there are better alternatives?

Then look at the general core principles of good health, such as diet, exercise and reducing stress, to see if simply by living better, you can remove these medications from your life once and for all.

When writing this chapter, I had tears in my eyes, as it served as a huge reminder of the false trust we place in doctors who we sadly think are acting in our best interests.

A lot of it is that doctors have been taught this in Med school and really believe it's the best thing for you, through no fault of their own, there is only so much that modern medicine can do and our local GP often doesn't have time to discuss alternative therapy. This makes it sadder, as these doctors do want to help, just for many of them they don't know how.

Your health is your responsibility. You cannot outsource overall responsibility to anyone.

Though you will at times need expert advice and guidance, ultimately, you need to be aware of what anything you put into your body will do and how it will affect you now and in the long term.

Your Action Plan - The Top 7 Medications That Cause Insomnia

This is not your typical action plan here, this is more an awareness that if in the future you are offered or even prescribed any of the below, you need to have a very serious chat with your health care practitioner.

In addition at this point I would suggest really upping your game when it comes to your health.

Then for those who are taking medicines, check that what you are taking is not on the below list and if so, I repeat the same advice as above.

1. Statins.

2. Beta blockers.

3. Alpha blockers.

4. Anti-Depressants.

5. Cholinesterase inhibitors.

6. Corticosteroids.

7. Antihistamines.

Your Personal Sleep Notes

"Sleep is the golden chain that ties health and our bodies together."

— Thomas Dekker

GET RID OF THAT PERSON NEXT TO YOU

13

This is big and one that really shocks people a lot!

People don't even think about how lying next to the person you love affects your sleep. We are so conditioned as a society, that it is completely automatic that you sleep every night in the same bed as your significant other.

Yet has anyone ever stopped to ask why we do this religiously?

Lying next to another human being has many disastrous effects on the quality of your sleep and, therefore, ultimately, how you feel the next day.

Huge Improvements in Your Sleep Quality

The quality of your sleep will improve massively as soon as you start sleeping alone.

When you first broach this topic you will be hit by fierce resistance and your partner may even think you have fallen out of love or it's something to do with them.

So, your first point of call is to make them understand it's nothing to do with them and is all about getting the best night's sleep possible. Reassure them and be supportive to their needs as it may come as a big shock to them.

To make this transition easier, explain to them why it's important to you. Most importantly, sell them the benefits, e.g. they get a more energised, calmer and kinder you. You will then have more energy to shower them with love and attention, what person could resist!

Give Your Partner a Wild Card

What I did to transition this and make the process a lot easier was to just make this a Sunday to Thursday sleep arrangement. Then come the weekends, I would share a bed. And to really spice things up, I would offer a "wild card", whereby once a month, she could bring out the said wild card, and we would spend the night together.

Or perhaps more conventionally, would be to start the evening together in bed whether this is for cuddles or other interesting activities, before you say your goodnights and retire to separate bedrooms.

Make it Bigger

If all else fails, the best option and an excellent option for those whose other bedrooms are taken up with children, is to buy a super king bed. This is a complete and utter game changer for you quite simply.

A bigger bed will allow you to put distance between yourself and your partner, while still allowing intimate and loving connections.

One of the significant issues I found when sharing a bed with my fiancé, was that she likes to strike out in the night and I would often be awoken to some random attack whilst she was in the midst of some exciting dream.

Stop Sleeping with Mike Tyson

Even if you don't have Mike Tyson sharing a bed with you, their movement throughout the night may drive some of you mad. Others who don't consciously notice this during their sleep will in fact, be taken out of your all-important deep sleep and REM sleep cycles - the really important quality part of your sleep.

You also have their hot body that will be heating you up, and one of the critical things for a great night's sleep is being cool, as the body's temperature drops when you sleep. Having another warm body next to you will raise your body temperature and reduce the quality of your sleep.

Separate Blankets

An excellent tip to combat this is to have separate duvets, which allows you to regulate your own personal temperatures better. Plus, no bitter midnight battles for duvet domination...

This is all before we even cover the obvious ones. Such as your partner bringing their phone into the bedroom with them and all the unwanted blue light that it brings, hitting your eyes and stimulating you. Just at the very time you want to sleep.

Your partner may like going to bed at different times than you so if you are the one going to bed first, they will wake you up when they get into bed.

Then if you are the one going to sleep first you will most likely be the one waking up first, in turn, waking them up when you get up.

Your Sleep Checklist - Get Rid of That Person

1. Does the person you sleep next to disturb you during the night, whether with constant movement, knocking you, snoring or stealing the blanket?

2. Does the person you sleep next to go to bed at a different time to you?

3. Does the person you sleep next to bring their phone or laptop to bed?

4. Does the person you sleep next to want a different room temperature or different thickness duvet than you during the night?

5. **Do you have a spare bedroom? If not, would a super king bed fit in your bedroom?**

_____

_____

_____

Your Action Plan - STOP Waking Up Tired.

1. Like everything we cover here in Sleep Mastery. Start slowly.

2. Perhaps start with doing this only one or two nights a week, before building it up to just weekdays and then spending the weekends together in bed.

3. Then if all else fails, get to the bed shop, and buy a super king bed with two sets of duvets.

Your Personal Sleep Notes

"Laugh and the world laughs with you, snore and you sleep alone".

— Anthony Burgess

IT'S NOT YOU, IT'S YOUR BEDROOM...

14

t is so ironic, that we call it a "bedroom" and yet, for most people, it's certainly more than that. It's a store of junk with clothes everywhere, entertainment systems like TVs and radios, and today even desks and computers make the cut as well. So, a bedroom has become not just a bedroom but an office, an entertainment room and a storage room, none of which is conducive for sleep!

One of the key things to getting a good night's sleep is turning your bedroom back into, well, a bedroom.

In this chapter, we will go over all the things in your bedroom that are doing the exact opposite of what a bedroom should be doing, allowing you to sleep soundly.

The Key Aspects of a Bedroom

Before we address the things stopping you from sleeping, let us outline what a bedroom needs to be for you to be a proper bedroom.

1. A cool room.
2. A humidity-balanced room.
3. A dark room.

4. A clear room.

5. A clean room.

When it comes to bed and bedding, this is a big subject and one I love, so I have written an entire chapter on this. Here though, I want the focus to remain separate from bedding and to consider the room itself.

This will allow you to focus, while keeping things really simple, so you can action as easily and quickly as possible for your great night's sleep.

A Cool Room

Though the ideal room temperature for sleep will vary on the individual and the type of bedding being used. Generally, a very good starting point for you is to get your bedroom to 19C/66F.

To ensure this, I have a thermometer in my bedroom to monitor the temperature close to bedtime.

Opening windows is one of the quickest and easiest ways to get the temperature down, and as a great bonus get some much needed fresh air into the house, that is of course, unless you live on a busy road, near airports, railway line, factories etc!

On hot days be aware that opening a window will only bring in hot air and in fact make your house warmer, particularly for south-facing rooms/windows. In this instance, simply wait until the evening to open and first thing when outside is nice and cool.

The same goes for your curtains and blinds, ensure throughout the day these are closed as they act as a great defence against the very powerful warming effects of the sun through glass.

For those of you in a polluted environment or who can't open your windows, e.g. penthouse apartment fifty storeys up, air conditioning is a must here.

Depending on what country you live in, this may mean you already have air con built into your property, which is typical in America, then you are good to go. For those in places like Great Britain, this will most likely require you to buy a mobile air-con unit. A good one can be bought for around $600/£500.

Humidity

This brings me nicely to another critical aspect of the room climate that nearly everyone overlooks - yet do this at your peril. Humidity!

Sleeping in too dry a room, under 40% relative humidity (RH), can cause problems such as:

- Increased risk of colds/flu.
- Dry eyes or irritable eyes.
- Flaky or itchy skin

While sleeping in too damp a room, over 60% RH, can cause problems such as:

- Feeling hot, bothered and sluggish.
- Mould, you really don't want this growing in any room, never mind a room you sleep in for eight hours a night.
- Heat stroke.
- Tiredness.
- Muscle cramps.
- Dehydration.

Personally, I like ALL my rooms in my house to be between RH 45% and 50%. However, I will only start taking action when my rooms go over 55%. As mentioned above, the quickest way is to open the windows or turn on the heating if too cold for an open window.

Now you are probably thinking, how the hell do I know what the humidity is in my house well simple! You get a hygrometer with a built-in thermometer. Two birds, one stone!

I have three of these around my house, one in the bedroom, of course, one in the living room and one in my office, which I am looking at now and is annoyingly 57%, time to open the window!

However, I also have a de-humidifier built into my mobile air-conditioning unit and these are brilliant. Mine will, in around 30 to 60 minutes, typically reduce humidity by 10%, taking the room from 57% to 47%, my sweet spot! This will of course depend on the model you invest in if this is an aspect you need to focus on.

Finally, while on the matter of what these air conditioning units can do, a lot of air-con units will have built-in air filters. These can take allergens such as pollen, dust mites, mould and chemicals from household products out of the air. Another great bonus, ensuring we breathe beautifully clean air.

A Dark Room

Now this one is easy.

When sleeping, your body likes darkness. It's that simple. We have loads of light sensors all over our bodies.

Firstly, the most important and powerful ones are those in your eyes, your melanopsin sensors. These help set your circadian rhythm.

They can detect what time of day it is by the corresponding type of light it's exposed to which changes throughout the day as the light goes from sunrise to sunset. In a nutshell, the melanopsin sensors tell your body when to wake up and when to sleep and it's for this reason that you want your bedroom to be a blackout zone.

Too much light in your bedroom at night will give your body mixed signals. Such as should I be asleep as even though I'm tired, there is still a lot of light…?

This is easy to fix. Depending on whether you have blinds or curtains, you can find a simple blackout option that goes on the back of your curtains on Amazon for $20/£15. In a matter of minutes, you have transformed your curtains from a source of light at night to pitch black.

Now I have also gone one step further. Again, this is simple and cheap to do. Light will still seep around the edges of the curtains even with these blackout curtains placed behind your existing curtains, so you want to tape the edges to ensure complete darkness.

A Clean Room

Your room should be clean. Any dirt and dust will be inhaled in varying quantities depending on how dirty your bedroom is.

Plus, having a clean room puts your mind at rest and makes for a relaxed sleeping environment conducive to a great night's sleep.

If you have cleaners, get them to pay particular attention to the bedroom as I know what cleaners can be like. They like to focus on the easy stuff like puffing cushions rather than the real job of cleaning!

Ideally, you want your bedroom being cleaned weekly, that's surfaces, hoovering/floors, cobwebs etc.

I appreciate this sounds basic; however, it's essential, so it needs to be addressed.

A Clear Room

Next, arguably one of the most overlooked yet essential aspects of a good night's sleep is a tidy bedroom, which means no clutter.

You want your brain to be as clear as possible, and if you got a huge stack of clothes piled up on the other side of the room looking you in the eye, this isn't going to happen. The brain is aware of it, even if you aren't!

Another thing that gets piled up in bedrooms is books. I have to be ruthless with myself on this one, with a maximum of two books at any one time. Though if one was going to be honest with themselves, this should be in fact be, just one book!

Ralph, you have been warned…

Toiletries do not belong in a bedroom; these are only the preserve of bathrooms!

TVs need to be thrown out the fucking window… NOW!

An absurd amount of fancy throws and silly pointless cushions, more clutter, get rid. Yes, I get it. The bed does look amazing; however, the bed can still look nice without all this pointless crap. It's just another thing to reduce your bandwidth.

Lots of shelves, you want your walls to be clear. Plus, the other big issue with shelves is that they attract junk that likes to be placed on them, which in turn generates more dust and more things to be maintained and cleaned.

I would go as far as to suggest that clothes, ideally, shouldn't be visible in your bedroom either. I personally have always used one of my other bedrooms for my clothes, though I appreciate it depends on the home layout and family dynamic as to whether that is possible. If your budget allows, built-in wardrobes are a fantastic investment. At the least ensure your clean clothes are in the wardrobe, and your unclean clothes are in the laundry basket - not in a pile to trip over in the morning!

You Sleep Checklist – Your Bedroom a Bedroom?

1. **Is your bedroom warm when you go to sleep?**

2. **Does light seep through your curtains or blinds, either through or around?**

3. **Is your bedroom cluttered and untidy?**

4. **Do you regularly have your windows open so that you have fresh air in your bedroom?**

Your Action Plan – STOP!! Waking Up Tired.

1. Set the temperature of your room to 19C/66F and experiment from there with the best temperature for you.

2. Install blackout blinds/curtains along with taping the edges.

3. Invest in a cleaner to clean your bedroom weekly.

4. Remove all clutter in the bedroom e.g. clothes, books, ornaments, shelves, and excessive cushions.

Your Personal Sleep Notes

"There is a time for many words,
and there is also a time for sleep".

— Homer

IT'S NOISY OUTSIDE

15

You might not be aware of the things that wake you up, it won't always be a loud bang of a neighbour's car door...

We wake up a lot during the night for several reasons, with external noises arguably the key, though this will very much be situationally dependent.

Historically and even now, we are at our most vulnerable when asleep, especially to attack as we can't defend ourselves.

In fact, I had a rather interesting encounter of just how vulnerable we are when asleep, having entered the world of dating again only last year. I was fast asleep in a date's bed and her ex-boyfriend from over a year ago - yes, over a year ago - came in, smashed me around the head with a kettlebell, then beat my head into the edge of the radiator next to the bed to give me the lovely scar I now have on my forehead.

However, annoyingly for me, we had Buddhist monks chanting Ohm rather loudly, sending us off to sleep, and this blocked out the noise, so I only awoke when covered in blood and he had left!

It's worth noting the woman I was with did leave an outside door open in her house due to the heat wave, foolishly knowing that she had a restraining order against her ex!

However, our bodies being the remarkable things they are, know there are dangers when we are asleep, so we have built-in systems that can alert us to any new dangers. With the loud Buddhist monks chanting in the background, this would sadly for me block out the noise and make me unaware of the dangerous threat to my life.

This is great that our bodies naturally alert us to these dangers even when asleep. Though in today's world where we live in our safe and secure houses, we in fact would benefit more from an environment free from external stimulation. One that the brain will not unconsciously focus on to determine if it's safe or not, with the odd exception such as a smoke alarm.

For this reason, we want to eliminate as much external noise as possible. In turn, our brainwaves can slow as much as possible.

Noise quite simply puts us on alert and wakes us up, whether consciously or unconsciously.

The 2 Main Sources of Noise that will Disrupt Your Sleep.

1. Internal noises that you can control.
2. External noises that you can't control.

Now I appreciate you do have some limited influence on certain external noises e.g. asking neighbours to be quiet, so you can certainly influence them or have some control. However, they also can tell you to piss off! Suppose it depends ultimately on your relationship with your neighbours and how nuts they are.

Internal Noises – The Noises You Can Control

Though I appreciate that this list won't be completely exhaustive, I am sure there are some "interesting" noises in your household that I don't know even exist!

The top ones include:

1. Dripping taps.
2. Noisy pipe work.
3. Creaking floorboards.
4. Draughty windows or doors.
5. Washing machines or dishwashers.
6. Loud TVs in other rooms.
7. Your partner and/or children are speaking loudly or making noise.

Luckily all of these can be managed and they don't cause a long-term problem. It's more about being aware that they exist and are a problem for your sleep. Then simply addressing them.

For things like taps and plumbing work, ensure all taps are always turned off tightly after use, which is standard anyway. Then for any more significant issues get a plumber in to fix them.

The same goes with any noisy floorboards, plus draughty windows and doors. If you can't nail it down yourself or simply don't want to get a carpenter to fix the issue.

Depending on the size of your house and where your washing machine is located relative to your bedroom, it might be necessary to only use during waking hours so as not to disturb any of you in the household.

Then when it comes to your partner or children's noise generation, ask them nicely to speak quieter and/or turn down their TVs.

If all else fails, remove their TVs, pocket money, credit card etc and turn the power off on a secure timer. Don't stand for any shit when it comes to your sleep, as it's the most important thing to protect for a great life.

External Noises – The Noises You Can't Control

Again though, I appreciate this list won't be completely exhaustive, as I am sure there are some "interesting" noises in your neighbourhood that I don't know about!

The top ones include:

1. Noisy neighbours.
2. Cars, trains and planes.
3. Drunk students and partygoers walking past.
4. Strong winds and storms.
5. Animals.

The Fan

This one is SO EASY!

In fact, one simple object will rectify nearly all of your noisy neighbour problems in one fell swoop – The FAN.

Yep, that's it, simply a fan.

"But how?" I hear you ask, can a fan stop all this; well, it is quite simple, as a fan will first block out nearly all background noise.

Secondly, big or loud noises are significantly reduced and, in most cases, muffled out, so they don't wake you up and have you begin the dreaded middle of the night falling back to sleep process!

Thirdly, if those two weren't enough, the white noise actually helps send you off to Lala land.

Finally, yes, there is even a fourth…the fan will also, would you believe, keep you cool at night. Hang on, isn't that what fans are for?

And we now know that the body loves a cool room to sleep in!

For Extreme Cases

There is very little you can do to actually reduce the output of noise from animals, strong winds, drunks singing, cars, trains or planes.

However, the solution comes in reducing its impact.

As already mentioned, the golden ticket is the fan. This will likely be the game changer that you need in your life.

However, for noises that operate on extreme levels, such as parties or planes flying overhead, first look at what you can control.

Can you install triple-glazed windows?

Can you put soundproofing in the walls, ceiling or floors of your bedroom?

Do earplugs work for you?

Personally, earplugs did absolutely nothing for me. However, they were recommended to me years ago by a friend combined with the fact that lots of places sell them, so perhaps they might work for you.

That being said, during the editing of this book my publisher spoke very highly of silicone ear plugs, that she has used for years to great effect. Though I haven't personally used silicone earplugs, based on her glowing review of them, these could be worth experimenting with as well.

As we are not all built the same, some things will work amazingly for one person, and for another, they won't move the needle one bit, so it's always wise to test different options for how they benefit you.

Always start with the things you can control.

When it comes to noisy neighbours, asking politely with respect wins hands down before resorting to threats and force.

And remember, you never fully know who you are dealing with…

Obviously, if things don't improve, you can become more forceful and/or involve the authorities. However, this can have a significant impact when it comes to selling your house, as you must declare all neighbourly disputes.

This could slow any future house sales down or impact the sale price. That's before we even cover the stress, which ironically will impact your sleep more than the noise itself!

Your Sleep Checklist – Shut the Fuck Up!

1. Is there any external noise at night that stops you from sleeping or wakes you up during the night i.e. neighbours, vehicles, animals or weather?

_____

_____

_____

2. Do you put on washing machines or dishwasher late at night that you can hear from the bedrooms?

_____

_____

_____

3. Do other inhabitants of your property generate any late-night noise?

_____

_____

_____

4. Does your property make noises, typically older properties will creek and their plumbing might not be as quiet as more modern properties?

_____

_____

_____

Your Action Plan – STOP!! Waking Up Tired.

1. Simply buy a fan.

2. If this doesn't drown out enough noise, buy a portable air-con unit, these are even noisier.

3. In really extreme cases where the other doesn't muffle out all noises and all else fails, invest in triple glazed windows and soundproofing of the walls, ceiling and floor, or if budget is a concern; order a decent pair or earplugs.

Your Personal Sleep Notes

"True silence is the rest of the mind, and is to the spirit what sleep is to the body, nourishment and refreshment."

— William Penn, Politician

CALM THAT BUSY MIND 16

One could argue that this is, in fact, the biggest killer of a great night's sleep in the Western world - a busy mind.

Some will call it stress. Others may even call it an overactive mind.

All true, and a huge problem if you want to sleep well and wake up performing your best tomorrow whilst also in a great mood.

This chapter will cover the best ways to remove stress from your life, though this will benefit your health and life in general.

The main areas for stress in most people's lives are:

1. Your thoughts.
2. Your work.
3. Your people.

I will go into each in detail as to why they annoy you and the best ways to remove this junk from your mind, ultimately it is only you they are harming!

Then I will unleash the nukes. This is like a powerful stealth weapon that many others, though they know it exists, don't fully realise the power this will have over you.

Your Thoughts – What Do You Think About?

If you are reading this the likelihood is that you are human, though obviously, I can't guarantee this! And if you are human, there is simply no way of avoiding stress altogether. We have to accept it as part of reality.

However, what I want this book to do for you, is not just reduce the stress you have, but to lower it to manageable levels, purely and simply to help you sleep better come night time!

Let's start with the quick, easy wins first.

The News

A super easy and quick win is to simply turn off the news. For those worried about the world and their country, this is one of the worst things you can consume.

Just turn it off!

Plus, you will also be very grateful for the time you save! Those into the news will watch it typically daily, and if you think 30 mins a day, which is easily done, works out at 900 minutes a month, which breaks back to 15 hours, or two average working days given back to you, every single month.

Now, who wouldn't want that amount of time given back to you?

Just think of how less stressful your life would be with all this extra time to get things done, plus you've also now recouped all the wasted time worrying about things you can't even control. That worry has now simply disappeared! A double whammy.

Focus on What You CAN Control

Following on from the news theme. Stop worrying about things in your life you can't control e.g. the state of the economy or terrorism and focus on what you CAN control.

This has a powerful effect on your mind. First, you no longer waste valuable time and energy on things you have little or no influence on, so they are best simply forgotten about.

Next, focusing on what you can control gives you a great sense of direction and a feeling of control in your life.

A Walk in Nature

This has to be one of my favourites. In fact, my second favourite and has worked time and time again, every time!

Do not underestimate the big impact on reducing your stress that simply going for a walk and being amongst nature can have on you.

Being by the sea, which is my favourite place to be when walking, provides you with lots of negative ions that are amazing for us, plus you hear the calming sounds of the sea.

Then there is the forest or mountains, whereby you get the phytoncide from trees and in Japan, it is even referred to as "forest bathing" due to all the goodness you get from nature.

Your Work – What Do You Worry About?

There are two amazingly simple and effective ways to reduce the effects of work-related stress.

These are:

1. Stop work at 7 pm, giving you a clear gap of between two and three hours before bedtime.

   This slows down and calms the mind before sleep. If I go past this time, I notice the difference when my head hits the pillow. It's just on overdrive…

2. I know I have mentioned this before, and I will say this again but put those bloody phones away!

Please turn off your phone, or at least put it on aeroplane mode an hour before bed. All the phone will do is alert you to new problems and worries that you didn't know about, which will in turn, make you more tired and grumpy come tomorrow - ironically when you want to be fresh and energised in the morning to deal with the issue properly.

Whereas now you won't be able to, as you had a shit night's sleep and will probably mess things up and make the problem worse with emotionally-led reactions.

Your People – Who Annoys You?

Let's be honest about this, without being true to yourself it's tough to make the changes you need and want. Trust me, I've been there!

If you find yourself angry multiple times a week and/or for long periods of time with a particular person you are going to struggle to sleep. No doubt about it.

Even if it's just one person! Never mind multiple people.

Why? These people will not just be on your mind. They will be on a continuous loop, going round and round in circles in your mind.

You have a few options to overcome this. Firstly, if this happens a lot and with numerous different people it's most likely you.

You can either deny it, as you are perfect and be in both long-term chronic pain AND then - it gets even better - be the most righteous man in the graveyard. OR, think "fuck having to be right all the time!".

As I'd rather feel happy and healthy all while seeing my great-grandchildren get married and have their first child!

However, there are times when you are simply surrounded by some of the most awkward, stubborn bastards this world has ever produced. I appreciate there are a lot of them out there!

I mention this in my book, STOP Killing Yourself…The Beginners Guide to Living Longer, that as much as I love my father very dearly; he sometimes, well, pretty much always, is such a man. Things like going out for a meal to putting new towels out when I stay, have caused huge arguments, and he is always right, of course!

So, be aware that some of the people you love most in the world can contribute to your early death…

In these cases, as I do with my dad, I only see him once a week now, he is my dad, and I love him very much. I can't, not see him, though often I will come away from seeing him, and my mood has changed for the worse. I feel the tension inside me and can even feel rather fucked off.

This is clearly not good for my health. So, I "remove" this toxicity from my life as best as I can, yet it's not easy I can grant you that!

Next we look at the people we have in fact personally chosen, friends, as some can be more like silent assassins than friends!

You will find that out of your group of friends, some people just cause problems, they attract them all the bloody time!

We all have had that one friend at some point (some of you still may have that friend and for some, you may even be that friend) that is a downer and sucks the joy out of life, always moaning or raring to go for an argument each time you see them. There are also the ones that take from you emotionally and physically. I had one and in the end realised that the friendship wasn't worth the cost on my mental health. I cut ties and haven't looked back since – was it easy? Maybe not initially, as I like to think I'm a nice person, but in the end I'm happier for it.

How Did You Get into My Life?

Now, if these are a colleague or a member of staff then it gets even more straightforward as you can quit or sack them! It may take a bit of time to manoeuvre your situation. However, it can be done and NEEDS to be done…soon!

Neighbours is an interesting one. You can be all chummy one day, then all of a sudden, for example, you don't mow your lawn when they want you to, of which I have first-hand experience of. The freak (man) who used to wash his car every single day, even if he hadn't been out in it for days!

Those twice-a-week, half an hour, pleasant conversations we always had suddenly turned into that same person completely blanking me. Now it took me weeks to work out the sudden split personality of the said neighbour opposite, and though still not sure, the mowing or lack of seems to be the most likely case…

Now I could confront him on this, which could quickly escalate into an argument and then all sorts of funny games to get one up on each other… Or as I have, you can simply ignore Jim Bob and carry on with a calm and peaceful life!

However, so many people refuse to let things go!

This is doing so much harm to your health. In fact, they are helping to stop you sleep. In turn contributing to killing you. So, each time you want to react, just remember, do you want them to slowly kill you?

It's worth noting he doesn't speak with his next-door neighbour either, so always a good move to spot these people early on as they can become your silent assassin if you choose to enter into their funny world of grudges and games…

Brain Wash Your Mind to Sleep

Another tactic I have developed is simply to just stop my mind from thinking of any thoughts. All I do is say SLEEP in my head as I breathe out, then remind myself that most thoughts discussed with me now will be forgotten come the morning, so I may as well not even bother wasting my time!

Plus, your only concern at this point is sleep. That's it, and that's by far the most important thing in your life at that moment.

Your Sleep Checklist – What Pisses You Off!

1. **Do you watch the news?**

    _____

    _____

    _____

2. **Do you work within two hours of bedtime?**

    _____

    _____

    _____

3. **Is your home/family/social life harmonious and relaxing?**

    _____

    _____

    _____

4. **Do you have a lot on your mind when you go to bed or does your mind become super active the moment you put your head on your pillow?**

    _____

    _____

    _____

Your Action Plan – STOP!! Waking Up Tired.

Only focus on what you can directly control, remove news and accept outside events you can't control. You worrying about them will do nothing to change them.

1. Go for a walk most days, ideally every day.

2. Do a review of everyone in your life and determine whether they add value to your life or do they bring you problems, then remove those problematic people.

Your Personal Sleep Notes

"I want to sleep but my brain won't stop talking to itself."

— Anonymous

IMPROVE
BYE, BYE ALARM CLOCK

SAME TIME TOMORROW... 17

We are so conditioned at what time we wake up that we have never even questioned whether this is the best course of action for us.

Well, it's not. Focusing on what time you go to sleep is far more important than focusing on what time you wake up. As you automatically set the scene for waking up at the best time for you and in effect when you want to.

When I am out, past my bedtime and my sleep alarms go off, people are both highly amused and baffled! Ralph, your alarm is going off. Oh, that's my 'first' alarm to go to sleep shortly, so I am going to have to leave in a bit.

They then say… "What you have an alarm to go to sleep? Are you nuts??"

It gets even funnier as that's not even the only alarm…

I have three alarms to go to sleep!

The first makes me aware that wherever I am, I need to be considering that it's bedtime soon, which is very handy when out as I will often get lost in conversation and forget all awareness of time. Also, if at home and reading, this signals that I can finish the chapter.

The next alarm is to inform me that I need to get into bed, put my book down and turn my phone on aeroplane mode now. Then, if out, a very grateful reminder that I haven't yet left where I am and need to leave now!

Then finally, as I like to read a book on mindset for the last half an hour of the day just before sleeping, this tells me it's lights out, Ralphy!

And lights out it is.

Then when morning comes, I have an incredible knack for waking up just before I want to, around 5.30am. I also have a backup alarm at 6am, for the occasional days I want a brief lie-in yet still want to seize the day.

Now, do I stick to this every single day of my life? Of course not!

Sometimes I simply can't be arsed, as I am human and will lie there if I have had a particularly demanding day, whether physically or mentally, until 8am and wrack up nine or ten hours of sleep!

However, most days, i.e. around six out of seven, this great habit kicks in and works wonders for my life.

One of the critical things when it comes to sleep, I have worked out over decades of optimising my sleep is that:

"Your tomorrow starts today."

And the best way to achieve this is... Same time tomorrow! Consistency of sleep time.

It doesn't stop there either. By setting a daily evening sleep routine, you get into great automatic habits of not just going to sleep but also telling your mind and body that you are in the process of going to sleep, making sleeping a lot easier and faster.

The easiest way to get great results is to build a habit and the easiest way to make a habit is to start small.

And arguably the MOST crucial sleep improvement habit or skill you could ever learn is:

"Go to bed the same time every single night."

The body loves this, as you get it into a familiar pattern, it knows when you do X. In my case, sauna at 7pm, sleep will soon follow.

So, let's look at my typical sleep plan every evening, which will help you see what I do. Then, we can run through each aspect and what you could do to make implementing this super easy.

Ralph's Evening Sleep Schedule

To help give you a real-life example, below is my winter sleep schedule. In the summer, when it gets dark around 10.30pm, I will often put back my sleep to 10pm simply because it just feels weird going to bed when it's still light. The key is to maintain a maximum of a thirty-minute window. Once you exceed this you put your body out of sync.

Whereas in the winter my sleep routine is consistently the below:

7pm – STOP!! Work Minimum Two Hours Before Sleep Time.

I want my brain to start to wind down and relax without having lots of busy thoughts radiating through my brain come lights out. Do not underestimate this aspect just because it sounds so simple.

7pm – Sauna, Walk or Socialise.

I tend to keep this a short walk so as not to over-stimulate the body and allow two hours between last exercise and sleep.

When it comes to sauna, I will have two 20 minute sessions, with a cold shower after the first and then a hot shower after the second so as not to stimulate myself too much.

8pm – Hot Shower & Pre-Sleep Ablutions.

There are a few reasons you don't want to wait until just before bed to brush your teeth, moisturise etc. The process of doing this, often overstimulates you and you often can't be bothered just before bed as you are tired. Plus, it will usually involve bright bathroom lights that will wake you up. The last thing we want before sleep is to overstimulate ourselves.

8.30pm – Read.

There is an argument that you should not read in bed and that your bed should simply be for sleeping. However, I like to read before sleep and I have trained my brain to recognise that reading will be the last thing I do before I fall asleep, therefore it has become part of my sleep routine and a habit.

9pm - Phone off and On Charge in Office.

We cover this shortly however, having your phone physically in another room stops you from getting out of that nice and warm cosy bed to go and blast yourself with blue light and mental stimulation.

9.30 pm - Lights Off and Sleep.

Let's now break each one down for you…

Set Your Alarm to Sleep

This is so important, as when creating a new habit you will sometimes forget and resort to autopilot. Which, in this case, is to go to bed after having worked late, come home from entertaining or having sat on the sofa watching TV all night etc.

Now, all I want you to do for the first day is set your alarm. In fact, do it now, get your phone out and set the alarm for the time you would like to go to bed.

You don't need to have any intention of actually going to sleep at this time. It's simply the time you would like to go to sleep every day.

Now for the next two days when the alarm goes off don't do anything (that's unless, of course, you want to). Just be aware for ten to twenty seconds that this is the new time you would like to start going to sleep at, then carry on with your evening.

On the third day, ask yourself, when the alarm goes off, are you ready to sleep now? If not, carry on with your evening.

Do the same on day four.

What Time Would You Like to Sleep?

By day five if you haven't started going to bed at this time already, I want you to take the time you usually go to bed against the time you want to go to bed.

For example, if you go to bed at 23.30 and want to go to bed at 22.00, then take 23.30 – 22.00 = 1 hour 30 mins.

Next, divide the time, in this case, 90 mins by 30, i.e. 3.

To change your sleep time by more than ½ hour a day is a challenging task for most people (not all, though), and my goal for you is your success. This requires you to put the best environment in place to facilitate your goals so that you action what you want to achieve.

So, in our example, it will take you three days (90 mins/30 mins = 3 days) to easily transition from 23.30 to your ultimate goal of 22.00.

Always remember small, simple steps every time. You want to make this easy on yourself.

Your Next Steps...

Would you like to wake up every morning and not feel guilty about having watched that 'extra' Netflix episode?

If so, this sounds like just the plan for you!

Waking up and feeling refreshed every morning is one of those beautiful yet simple life gifts and it's one I love to share to help people.

Please be aware that I am no saint, and I do from time to time also stay up late watching films and have the occasional lie-in. This is not to be a rigid iron-clad plan, but more a structure or basis for how to build a life and life is there to break the rules from time to time.

Your Sleep Checklist - What Are Your Timings?

1. What time do you go to bed and what time would you like to go to bed?

2. Do you wake up the same time every day, including weekends?

3. Do you get a good dose of natural light first thing in the morning?

4. Do you have an alarm for bedtime or have an evening bedtime routine?

5. **Does your partner or children stop you from going to bed when you want?**

Your Action Plan – STOP!! Waking Up Tired.

1. Write down the time you go to bed and wakeup typically.

2. Write down the time you would like to go to bed and then set the alarm on your phone to this time every evening.

3. Calculate the optimal number of days this is going to take for you to transition to your new sleep time.

4. Make it happen by planning an evening sleep routine that increases your chances of this happening most nights.

5. Find out the best time for you to wake up.

Your Personal Sleep Notes

"Legend says that when you can't sleep, it's because you're awake in someone's dream. So, if everyone could stop dreaming about me, that would be great."

— Anonymous

THE BEST LONGEVITY MACHINE IN THE WORLD

18

Hang on Ralph, a bed, we all got those, that's nothing new, surely?
It was only when I started writing my guides to the world's best longevity machines back in 2020 that I realised the bed is in fact the best longevity device in the world!

If it's not, then I can't think of a better one at this moment in time and I used to sell longevity machines!

It dawned on me that we need to think of the bed not as a piece of furniture but as a longevity device, and not just any but the most important longevity device you can ever buy.

So, without further ado, let me explain why this might be the most important thing you ever buy. Even more important than your house…

When it comes to your bed, there are so many factors to consider which is why in this chapter we are going to break back all the aspects into one simple place for you to understand. You will know what to look for in order to make your bed - the best longevity device in the world.

The Key Issues of Modern Beds

1. Materials that are toxic to humans are often used in their construction.
2. Ventilation is often non-existent causing us to overheat and lie in our own sweat.
3. Lack of support creates back problems and pain.
4. Horizontal sleeping position are a problem because your brain rejuvenates best when sleeping at a slight incline.

What Your Bed Consists Of?

The three areas of concern when it comes to what your bed is made of are:

*   The bedframe.
*   The mattress.
*   Any metals used.

Just Like your Food...

Just like your food you want your bed to be made from natural organic materials.

This means natural hard woods, using organic oils to give you a great finish. Not synthetic materials, paints or varnishes. These give off gas due to their volatile organic compounds (VOCS).

Ultimately this means, you are sleeping on top of a chemical cesspit, giving off toxic gasses, polluting your bedroom's air supply and therefore the air that you breathe in for eight hours every night!

Your Mattress

Next is the mattress,. What's yours filled with?

We want to avoid polyester plus other synthetic materials, and especially petroleum chemical-based foams. These foams can take the form of being both a memory foam mattress, or used in addition to springs as a mattress topper.

An interesting angle on the "natural" marketing of beds are mattresses advertised as natural or as sustainable horsehair, since these are in reality treated before construction of your bed in yet another chemical process.

We often see flame retardants advertised as a positive. However, these are just laden with toxic chemicals. Again, no thank you.

Metal. This is something frustratingly I only found out months after buying my super luxurious and amazingly comfortable super king mattress at a cost of $2,500 (£2,000). And yes, I am struggling to part company with it, however in time I will, just not yet!

Metal has long been proven to interfere with our quality of sleep, in particular our natural sleep rhythm. The majority of mattresses are spring based, and what are springs made out of? Lots of metal.

Though not common, some people, especially the elderly, who ironically will be most affected by this, have electrically adjustable beds. These electrical motors are just oozing out EMF radiation, right next to you all night long just without the beautiful voice of Lionel Richie!

Ever Slept With Sweaty Betty?

Now don't get me wrong, sweating is a natural part of everyday life and especially when we sleep, as it's part of our detoxification process. Think the sweats after a heavy boozing session!

However, we don't really want to be woken up continuously due to wet patches of sweat, do we now?

The best way to overcome this is to have a bed and mattress that allows your skin to breathe at night and in turn allow the sweat to naturally evaporate, as opposed to soaking into your sheets.

The key aspects of whether your sweat evaporates, leaving you dry and importantly asleep or wet and awake and not in a fun way, is your mattress, bed and bedding.

We will be covering bedding in the next chapter. This chapter is just focusing on your bed itself.

You want your bed to have under-bed ventilation i.e. fresh air should flow underneath your mattress and bed which helps cool you from underneath.

The other key benefit of a dry bed is that you don't attract uninvited guests to sleep with you, such as those lovely dust mites, mould and bacteria.

Your Sleeping Partner Not Being Supportive These Days?

No not your actual partner, your bed!

As a man in my 20s, I would regularly experience new beds and it would often dawn on me, what uncomfortable contraptions a lot of them were. Whether they had springs digging into me or that they completely lacked support.

This would lead to me being disturbed throughout the night and in turn waking up feeling rubbish the next day. This was in addition to the new and most unwelcome stiffness the next day.

It is hardly surprising when you think about it, we are on our, or someone else's, bed for eight hours every day. This is a third of our lives, so if anything is going to have a big impact on your body's infrastructure, it's going to be your bed.

Closely followed by your working position, i.e. for most of us our desk and chair!

A bed can do one of three things for you.

Where you had no problems or aches previous to this new bed, it can now create such problems and aches for you.

If you already have posture issues, it can make them a lot worse for you.

Or it can improve your posture and relieve back pains. Rarely is a bed neutral, generally it's either helping your posture or making it worse.

I have done multiple tests of sleeping on the floor. Yes, the hard cold floor! I wanted to experience first-hand how my back felt after sleeping on such a hard surface.

The first two or three nights you find you wake-up a lot, as your body can't quite understand why the surface you're sleeping on is so hard and it doesn't have any give and move like your mattress.

This leads to continuously waking up throughout the night, which obviously is not good for your sleep for the first two or three nights. However, you do wake up with this lovely and completely revived body posture, something that's hard to explain in words. Though very welcome and invigorating.

Once you have overcome the first few nights, something magical happens - you get used to this new hard surface while also benefiting from a rejuvenated body.

Do I sleep on the floor every night? Of course not. There needs to be a balance. This led me to look into different sleep systems or beds as most people call them.

Sleep Like You Are Japanese

One of those was the Japanese method of sleep.

This was a step up from my floor method, thankfully! It consists of having a mat as the foundation, often directly on the floor, called the Tatami Mat. Next "the mattress", which is essentially a topper over the Tatami mat, called a Shikfuton, which is made from cotton.

Then, what we would call a duvet, the Kakefuton, is filled with silk fibres which are great for even heat distribution and a hostile environment for dust mites, exactly what us humans want!

However, by being on the floor, as covered above, you are not allowing for ventilation underneath you as you sleep, plus you are close to dust and other allergens whilst that low to the ground.

When you sleep, you want your back supported in the right places, which is simply to maintain the spine's natural shape, yes that simple!

You want your natural S-shaped curvature of your spine supported, with even distribution of pressure. Which as I found out when sleeping on the floor for two weeks, though very supportive, I could feel a lot of pressure around my hips/lower back area.

Another heavy area of our bodies that have an impact on pressure and your muscles, are your shoulders. This causes us to lose the natural shape of our spine in a lot of mattresses. Of course, our muscles then overcompensate to alleviate this and maintain balance, however this is what creates your back pain and tension.

The Angle of Your Bed

This one is going to blow your mind, as it did mine, when I first discovered this many years ago!

The best way to sleep is with your head slightly above your feet. Yes, this means that the traditional way of us sleeping lying flat, is not the best way for you.

The solution, have the top of your bed i.e. your head end, around 3-6 inches higher than the bottom end of your bed i.e. where your feet are. The aim is to get an elevation of around 3-5 degrees.

This has to do with the world's most popular cause for dis-ease, inflammation, which is a result of a build up through the day (and your life) of toxins.

Our bodies have amazing ways to deal with these toxins or waste products of the body, it's called the lymphatic system, which I am sure you've heard of. Then for your brain, we have the glymphatic system, which is the brain's equivalent of the lymphatic system.

By sleeping at an incline and simply taking advantage of gravity, this helps promote your brain's glymphatic system and in turn remove toxins from it, all while you are fast asleep.

Why is this important? Well, 90% of your brain's detoxification occurs while you are asleep. In particular deep sleep, that time when if someone wakes you up you are disorientated and drowsy.

Other benefits include, reduced snoring, reduced sleep apnoea and less heartburn! Talk about multiple wins from one simple change.

Which is why sleeping at an incline is such a big game changer in your life, with better health, a better brain and you also get to live longer!

Dust Mites & Bed Bugs

Even if you don't suffer from allergies, these will affect your sleep for the worse. Why? As the little bastards will be biting you and you can be awoken from deep sleep by the itching, which in my opinion, is more annoying than the actual bite.

What is more annoying than being woken up by some creature biting you in the dark?

For those with allergies it doesn't even bare thinking about, as not only will you be woken up, but you also most likely won't go back to sleep like the rest of us straight away. In fact, you will probably just lie there itching yourself with red eyes, all whilst sneezing a lot due to how good these little buggers are for setting off people's allergies.

Bed bugs just love our human skin. Not sure why anyone would be surprised as I like my human skin as well! We shed around six grams of dead skin a week, so where better to live, than in your bed!

Plus, they also like a warm moist environment, so they just don't get a double whammy, they get a triple whammy of juicy benefits by sleeping with you!

This is why it's always a great idea to have a warm shower, not a cold shower which will energise you before bed. Plus a warm shower helps you sleep better, never mind that beautiful feeling of clean skin against clean sheets!

Then have both a bed that's well ventilated and in a well-ventilated room, so think windows open and keep humidity between 45% to 50%.

You want a bed that allows fresh air to aerate up from underneath, yes that means ditching those amazingly handy under bed draws. I've had them and yes, they are an amazing use of space, however your health and therefore your sleep is much more important than having a nice place to store your bedding!

Having an open bed frame is the best way to do this. It's also worth noting that warm metal spring coils can attract bed bugs and if that wasn't bad enough, also mould!

So, the very place you think you are going to repair and rejuvenate your body and mind every night is in fact potentially making you ill.

Your Sleep Checklist - Your Sleep Infrastructure

1. Do you know what materials your bed is made out of?

2. Is your mattress made of foam or metal springs?

3. Does your bed allow for underneath ventilation?

4. Is your bed supportive, or is it too soft or too hard?

5. **Do you think you may have bed bugs i.e. do you often get bits and itches?**

Your Action Plan – STOP!! Waking Up Tired.

1. Due to both the attachment and cost of one's bed, I am not saying to throw your bed away and get one that does everything as listed above. Though that would be good and by all means if you have the funds, then please do so.

2. What's best in this instance is that if your bed is old, then now is a great time to use this new found knowledge to get a real good bed for you.

3. For those of you who have just bought a bed or really like their bed like me, then make some of the changes. Perhaps you could keep the mattress and change the bed frame, then put your old bed in the guest room or give it to one of the kids?

Your Personal Sleep Notes

"*Me: Please let me sleep! Brain: Nope, we have to stay up together and go over every bad life decision we have made so far.*"

— Anonymous

BE CAREFUL WHAT YOU
TOUCH AT NIGHT

19

This is a very underestimated and often overlooked aspect of a great night's sleep and a morning bursting full of energy. So, let's point you in the right direction.

When it comes to your bedding, you have three aspects of improving:

1. The pillows.
2. The duvet.
3. The sheets.

Keep it Real

The fabric choice of your bedding is key. Natural fibres win hands down over synthetic polyesters, nylon and chemical-based foams etc.

Natural fibres include cotton, linen, silk and wool.

On this topic, I want to give you my personal experience, as this will give you a better insight and relate to your situation more than just telling you what you should get.

When it comes to sheets, I have always gone for the very finest Egyptian cotton and silk sheets. I love the contrast between the two as they are so very different, yet both are so magical to sleep with.

When it comes to your pillow and duvet filling, I've always slept with feathers, Siberian Down in particular, arguably the best feathers in the world or at least a close second to Canadian Goose.

Though arguably one of the best bedding fabrics, sadly, I have yet to experience it first-hand myself, this being organic wool. When I next come to change my bedding I will replace it with organic wool.

Should I be throwing out my feathers today and buying organic wool now? Yes, however, I can't quite bring myself to throw away my very expensive and very comfortable bedding, just yet.

I've learnt in life that the key to getting into world-class habits is a process of slowly but surely. Nothing too drastic, and your ego will agree to it. Otherwise, your ego will resist and self-sabotage even the best-laid plans!

As I do everything else that I write about when it comes to mastering my sleep, there's the odd thing I can live with. Though if I were earning a few million a year, I would be more inclined to treat my bed and bedding as sunk costs and move forward with a Samina bed and organic wool bedding.

Your Pillows

For a very long time now, the only pillows I have slept with have been some of the finest Siberian Down feathers in the world. These have been great for me over the years.

They are natural, so there is no off-gassing from artificial chemicals, they are incredibly comfortable, and I sleep very well.

A few years ago I wanted to test out natural silk pillows from my favourite bedding supplier during the start of lockdown, so I ordered a set and waited extremely patiently yet very excitedly for the big day to arrive.

Sadly the big day never came for me to put silk and feather pillows head-to-head (get it!). King of Cotton, who have been supplying me with fantastic quality bedding and service for 15 years had annoyingly ran out. Even more infuriatingly they have now since discontinued their Mulberry silk.

I'll get to try them soon hopefully and I'll update a second edition to let you know!

The Shape of Your Pillow

The main purpose of a pillow is to support your neck and in turn align your spine.

When people think of pillows they mainly think of what they are made out of. However, we also need to be thinking of a pillow's shape as well.

Aside from the standard rectangle-shaped pillow, there are two new shapes I want to introduce you to.

The first being almost like a U-shaped valley. This is raised at the point where the pillow meets your shoulder to support the neck, then dips where your head goes.

Perfect for those side and back sleepers.

Then, perhaps the most interesting option of them all… the Body Pillow. This allows one pillow to take care of neck support, somewhere comfortable to support your hands and critically a great way to support your spine by going between the knees.

Your Duvet

Like my pillows, I have for decades been a big fan of feathers!

It all started many years ago when I dated a girl, well more like a woman when I was 25, and she was 34. I remember the first time I stayed at hers, she had the most incredible bedding. I exclaimed the very moment I awoke from that first night staying at hers, *"why is your bed so amazing!?!"*

She replied, "feathers darling, it's all about the feathers darling!"

Later that day, when I was back home the first thing I did was of course go feather hunting!

To this day it was one of the best things I ever did. The comfort and delightful sleep I can attribute to my feathers are incredible!

However, that being said there is a new kid on the block and it doesn't tweet, it baahs!

We touched on organic wool above and what makes wool so amazing Ralph? I can hear you asking… well first up, it can absorb up to a third of its own weight in moisture, which makes it great for those sweaty Bettys!

While its hollow fibres help keep an even temperature under the duvet for you. Regulation of your sleep temperature is critical to a great night's sleep. Excess heat will keep you from falling asleep and will wake you up throughout the night.

Plus, I have my famous little trick on how heat is a fantastic way to wake you up in the morning, though that requires setting your heating and has nothing to do with your duvet.

Also, remember that as the seasons change so will your duvet potentially. For me, I use the same duvet all year round, as I have an air conditioning unit in my bedroom that in the summer keeps my bedroom at the same constant temperature my heating does in the winter.

So, bear this in mind throughout the year based on your bedroom's climate control.

Your Sheets

As with most things, and especially like your partner, you want them natural!

Of course, your bed sheets are no different. It's for this reason a great place to start is with organic Egyptian cotton with a minimum thread count of 400g per square meter.

If you have polyester sheets or any other synthesized fabrics, then please simply throw them out. Yes, I will repeat that. Throw them out.

If you are feeling really flush, then why not go for 1,000 thread count which I treated myself to a few years ago and this, combined with the best feathers in town, makes night-time a dream, quite literally...

I also have 400g/m2 as though the 400g/m2 doesn't compare to the 1,000g/m2. The contrast is really nice to have, as you appreciate the difference. Plus, when it comes to summertime heat waves, you will be glad for the lighter and thinner 400g/m2.

In addition to this, I also have silk sheets mainly for summer, though they will be brought out a few times during winter as well, and they are the pinnacle of luxury and a great night's sleep. Though interestingly, you tend to lose a pillow during the night as the silk is so slippery!

Bio-ceramic Organic Wool

A manufacturer who I admire (if you ask me I'll tell you who) offers a very special bedding combination of 60% organic cotton and 40% bio-ceramic yarn sheets that includes various minerals and crystals. This is then all wrapped around virgin sheep wool to create soft and supple mattress toppers, pillows and duvets. This natural bedding optimally balances heat and moisture for a dry and warm bed.

In addition to this, the Bio-ceramic fibres help promote detoxification and relaxation and reduce stress on the body. All of these help for a deeper sleep and more energy and a better mood come morning.

Your Sleep Checklist - Whose Sharing Your Bed?

1. What are your pillows and duvet made from?

2. What materials are your sheets and pillowcases made of?

3. Do you find your bedding too hot in the summer or too cold in the winter?

4. Would you benefit from different shaped pillows to help support your neck, back or legs better?

Your Action Plan – STOP!! Waking Up Tired.

1. Keep it real. Ensure that you have natural bedding only and preferably organic.

2. Look into different shaped pillows as they may serve you better than traditional rectangle, one size fits all?

3. Is your duvet the right level of warmth for you? You are after Goldilocks, not too hot nor too cold!

Your Personal Sleep Notes

"Each night, when I go to sleep, I die. And the next morning, when I wake up, I'm reborn."

— Gandhi

TIME TO RELAX 20

A few game changers to ensure you relax come the evening, these are:

1. Bright lights.
2. Bath & showers.
3. Music.
4. Meditate.

Bright Lights

I appreciate we have already covered a dark room in the chapter on your bedroom. However, this is a very different angle, though the same theme.

First off, exposure to bright lights before even entering bed is detrimental to your sleep that night.

For this reason we need to ensure that around 7pm the lights in the house are dimmed or turned off.

I mentioned in earlier chapters about using lamps or lights in other rooms to help reduce your exposure to bright light.

When you go to bed only have your bedside lamp on which will be a very low-level light, just enough to read yet not too bright to wake you up.

And this one is a biggie. Get rid of bright solid spot lights in your bathroom. If you must have them, fit a shaving light for evening use. No shaving required! This is a lot dimmer for evening use and won't stimulate you too much.

Bath and showers

The key question here is, hot or cold?

Many people think a cold shower is a good idea to help them sleep, and for some it might. However, for most people it's not. What you in fact want is a warm to hot shower or hot bath.

The reason is quite simple when we sleep, our internal temperature drops, which is why you find it so hard to sleep during a heat wave like we are currently experiencing as I write this book.

So, the best way to cool your internal body temperature, would you believe it, is to in fact have a hot shower and not a cold shower. Bizarre…

However, when you think about it, think back to how you feel after a cold shower. Super stimulated and ready for action!

So, what's the last thing you want to be when going to sleep? Of course, super stimulated, that's why a cold shower for most people should not be had just before bedtime.

That being said, I have heard of people who say it works for them, so by all means try it however, for most people a warn shower will work far better.

Music

I don't want to spend too much time on music, as tastes are very individual. However, listening to happy hardcore rave music just before sleep, even for the hardest raver, is not going to set you up for a great night's sleep.

On the flip side, pretty much anyone, even if they don't like soft relaxing classical music, will benefit from the relaxing and soothing sounds before bed.

If you struggle with relaxing and sleeping, experimenting with different types of calming music, and the key word here is calming, will yield great results.

Meditation

One of my favourites, and one of the most significant habits I have learnt in my life, has been to meditate daily.

The benefits overspill into so many other areas of your life. It's, in fact, quite unbelievable, and while this is a sleep book, I strongly recommend you try. I am extremely grateful for how much calmer and relaxed I am in general day-to-day life as a result.

Perhaps it could do the same for you?

It's very rare I lose my temper these days and it's directly correlated to meditation.

Now, my key reason for bringing up mediation, is of course to help you sleep.

Before you do what I did, let me give you a bit of insight. About five years ago when I first decided to meditate, as the great Ray Dalio recommended, I got very confused as to what I had to do and would 'try' to meditate, when in fact it's really simple.

I will give you a brief crash course in creating brilliant habits and show you how you can begin the amazing habit of daily meditation.

Think SMALL, in Fact, VERY SMALL

The reason most people never start anything is that they get overwhelmed.

It's too much!
How am I ever going to find the time to do that?
How am I ever going to learn how to do it?

Want the good news? Of course you do…

Well, start off with the simplest and most basic version of what you want to achieve to begin with.

With no pre-conceived ideas, simply see if it works or not. Don't worry about whether you're doing it right. Just do it and do the smallest unit possible.

The best way to explain is with an example. I will use a personal example of me 'trying'" to start meditating for a number of years of, which I now do every day for half an hour and an hour on Saturdays and Sundays.

Yet ironically my goal was only twenty minutes on weekdays!

However, it didn't start like the picture-perfect routine others see daily. Hell no, I tried for years to meditate.

I would get into a right pickle. I would make up silly excuses why I couldn't do it. I would make up more important things to do, like stack the dishwasher or check emails!

Yeh, these things are so much more important than mediating, aren't they Ralph? Then there was the fact that I was confused about what to do having been given so many conflicting ways to meditate.

Then one day I just decided that I didn't know what I was doing and that was ok and I would just start meditating. So, I did. I simply sat down on the floor with my back against my sofa. I placed my hands in my lap, put my legs in a position where the soles of my feet were touching as I find being crossed legged rather uncomfortable.

The real key to begin with was that I decided NOT to do twenty minutes which was my end goal, I just did one minute!!!

YES, can you believe I went to all the effort to sit comfortably for just ONE minute of meditation?

Now here comes the real key thing, I didn't do just one minute of meditation, now did I, even though that was the plan? I thought, well, as I am here, I may as well carry on as it's not that bad and if I'm honest, I am actually quite enjoying it. I ended up doing three minutes.

So, I trebled my plan and finally for the first time in my life, I got round to meditating.

Over the course of the next few days I set myself a small goal and each day I exceeded it. Within a very short time I had actually attained half of my ultimate end goal.

Then over the next week, I went from ten mins to fifteen and then finally to twenty, my ultimate end goal, and that was all achieved in just two weeks after five years of pissing about and procrastinating.

Your quick takeaway is:

"ALWAYS start SMALL and SIMPLE!"

"Set NO expectations on the outcome."

Your Sleep Checklist - Time to Relax

1. Do you have the house lights on full during the evening up to the point of bedtime?

2. Do you meditate?

3. Do you watch action, drama, or horror programs in the evening?

4. Do you have a warm shower or bath before bedtime?

5. **Do you listen to loud and/or energic, heavy metal, rave or similar music late at night?**

Your Action Plan – STOP!! Waking Up Tired.

Turn off or dim all lights in your house around two to three hours before bedtime.

1. Have a hot shower or bath before bed to cool down your inner core, plus it makes you feel so much cleaner and cosier in bed.

2. Start meditating for just one minute a day.

Your Personal Sleep Notes

"Many things — such as loving, going to sleep, or behaving unaffectedly — are done worst when we try hardest to do them."

— C. S. Lewis, Studies in Medieval and Renaissance Literature

YOUR FAVOURITE POSITION? 21

When it comes to one of the most impactful aspects of your sleep, we don't have a huge array of choices. In fact, we have just three options and they are:

1. On your front.
2. On your back.
3. On your side.

Preference over Science

There will be an element of personal preference regardless of the scientific research, it will take you at least a week to really get used to a new sleep position. The first few nights your body is not used to this new position and it will want to go back to what it's familiar with. In turn you will wake numerous times throughout the night.

A month is a good minimum to try these things properly. Yes, I know it's a long time. However, we are talking about the rest of your life here, not some restaurant for the evening!

The first few nights of a new sleep position for some, though not all, can be challenging, as you automatically want to go back to what you are used to and it can be a mental fight. Trust me, I've been through it a few times.

Oddly as I write this, it's been a terrible heat wave here in the UK. Even with air conditioning it's still been a little tough, so I have noticed that to comfort myself I have caught myself multiple times resorting back to my long-term sleeping position that I changed a few years ago!

It's interesting that habits I changed and mastered years ago have resurfaced their ugly head during times of resistance. It's the same to be fair of most bad habits. The human brain is very clever and interesting, that's for sure.

Ultimately, if you get a great night's sleep in your preferred position, don't change it. As the old saying goes, "if it ain't broke, don't fix it!"

Only do so if you feel things could be better, as you will have to experience at least a week of broken sleep getting used to your new sleeping position.

The Best Sleeping Position

The reason it's so key to get a great sleeping position is that it can be the difference between a great night's sleep and no sleep!

Plus, the impact on muscles and joints is crucial. How often over the years have you woken up with brand new aches and pains that didn't exist yesterday? No prizes for guessing where they came from!

A big aim of "STOP!! Waking Up Tired" is to ensure you never wake up again with such aches and pains. Everything we do in "STOP!! Waking Up Tired" is to optimise your tomorrow and not just tomorrow's tomorrow, but every tomorrow's tomorrow.

If you are waking up in pain, whether minor or severe, you are not performing at your best that day. As with all the chapters in the book my aim is to get you to perform at your best every single day.

This is why it's essential to understand that certain sleep positions can help relieve stress on your spine, while others can in fact increase pain in your neck, shoulders, back and arms while you sleep.

As mentioned, this is not a one size fits all, however the common theme is all about a sleep position that supports a healthy spine alignment for you. That being said, there are widely supported positions that are best for the majority of people and we are going to cover those now.

On Your Front (Stomach)

I absolutely loved sleeping on my stomach until a few years ago. In addition to this bad habit, I would also have my arm under my pillow, which would mean that come 3am I would wake up with intense pins and needles in my arms if I were lucky or, more likely, a numb arm!

This is a horrible way to be woken. Though it wouldn't happen every night, it did happen enough that it needed to be changed, no matter how much I liked lying on my stomach. Like with changing any habits, I started slowly.

The ultimate aim was to sleep on my side. I started off still sleeping on my stomach for a few nights, though this time placing my arm to the side of me, against staunch opposition from my mind, though still on my stomach. Then after a few nights, I was able to progress to the ultimate end point of sleeping on my side. Which six and a half nights out of seven I now do.

Though I have the odd relapse, interestingly these relapses are when I am not paying attention and as soon as I realise, I will correct my sleep position. Without knowing the crafty brain can put you in that position, so be aware of the unaware!

For most of us sleeping on your side is best for supporting your spine, as it places less pressure on your spine. Followed by sleeping on your back.

For me, I originally found this hard to believe being a staunch stomach sleeper, and in fact I occasionally relapsed to a front sleeper. Interestingly this is the least most popular sleeping position amongst us humans.

The significant issue I found with sleeping on my stomach was that my neck would have to twist for me to breathe and not have my face down, suffocating into my pillow! This would give me occasional neck aches which I am sure fellow front sleepers will have also gotten from time to time.

The other issue I had with front sleeping was that I was putting pressure on my rib cage; therefore, this would impact my breathing to some degree. Though, of course, this will vary tremendously among individuals due to weight, your shape and the exact position you sleep.

Then finally, front sleeping also provides the least support for your back i.e. increasing pressure throughout the night on your spine.

Going back to my aesthetic days, I would also practice getting myself to sleep on my back to reduce the effect of wrinkles, as just as lying on your side, you are crunching up your face for many hours every night.

Generally, lying on your stomach is the worst sleeping position you can adopt or maintain. For this reason I suggest, like I have had to do, you practice sleeping on your side and if that's not any good try sleeping on your back.

If you really, really must insist on your stomach, then it's critical that your mattress is firm and through much testing of ways to improve sleeping on my stomach, I found that only using one pillow was better than two pillows, which raised my head too high.

Another great piece of advice for front sleepers who don't want to change is that having my legs out to the side, with a pillow between my knees, worked wonders for me. So more of a hybrid sleeping position, as I am at a 45-degree angle as opposed to flat out on my front.

For most of us, sleeping on your side is best for supporting your spine, as it places less pressure on it. Followed by sleeping on your back.

On Your Side

Most people sleep on their side. Around 60% of people, even more so for males. So, if most people are already doing this, that means there is not much else to do for most of you when it comes to sleeping positions! Which is excellent news.

As we get older, our spine flexibility reduces which makes sleeping on your side more supportive and comforting for older people, which makes it great for those with back pain.

Plus, it's also great for reducing snoring, acid reflux and heart burn. Though sleeping on your side can increase your wrinkles.

A few issues with sleeping on your side, namely shoulders. So, if you have shoulder issues, this might not be your best sleeping position due to the extra pressure you are focusing on this one area.

Though it might be just a case of swapping up positions throughout the night. changing between side and back, this way giving you the best of both worlds. Which is what I do, to minimise facial wrinkles and excessive pressure on my body of any one particular spot.

Left is the New Right

Would you believe there is a best side to sleep on! When I found this out years ago I found it somewhat amusing however it does make logical sense.

Sleeping on the left is best for you, as sleeping on your right increases the pressure on your internal organs. Plus, the way your intestines are laid out internally, left side sleeping allows for a more efficient clearing out of your system!

I would argue this is even more important and therefore beneficial for you. Sleeping on your left side also has a very interesting benefit when it comes to living longer with a sharper brain. Due to a better clearing out process overnight of your mental garbage that accumulates in your brain throughout the day called interstitial waste.

On Your Back Love

Now we come to the world's second most popular position.

As you can imagine it's the obvious choice for supporting your spine and evenly distributing your body weight as lightly as possible.

Aim to keep both hands in the same or at least similar positions to distribute pressure evenly on your spine. Plus this also helps with your overall weight being evenly distributed.

Developing on this theme, lying on your back is also best for those with neck pain. Think of the position of your neck twisted when on your stomach. Or the potential for your neck to either drop or be too highly elevated on your side.

Feather pillows work well for supporting your neck, as they allow the heavy head to sink, while the pillow supports the lighter neck. Other options typically suggested include memory foam. However, we don't want to use memory foam due to the chemicals used to make the foam.

If you feel the feather pillow is not enough to support your neck, try a simple towel rolled up or other household items that can provide the desired level of support for your neck.

Also, as alluded to many times before with my skin clinics, I loved lying on my back for the lack of effect it causes my facial skin and therefore wrinkles.

For you snorers out there, you of course know this is the worse sleeping position for your snoring and you certainly will know if your partner snores that this is the worst position for them, as well as you!

The same goes for acid reflux and sleep apnoea. However, if you have these, you will already know this, well you do now!

Then finally, a note to those heavier than they should be and those getting older, it becomes harder to breathe when lying on our backs due to the pressure of gravity.

Your Sleep Checklist – Your Best Side Forward

1. What's your favourite sleeping position?

2. Do you wake up with any stiffness or aches?

3. Do you use pillows for support between your legs?

4. Do you have a bad back?

Your Action Plan – STOP!! Waking Up Tired.

1. If you are sleeping on your stomach, then from tonight start practising with either sleeping on your side or back. Both have benefits and which is best can often be down to the individual.

Your Personal Sleep Notes

"The amount of sleep required by the average person is five minutes more."

— Wilson Mizener

YOUR PERSONALISED SLEEP PLAN
SLEEP MADE EASY FOR YOU

SUMMARY

22

Simply having read this book, you have taken in a lot of new information. You are now aware of a new world, that perhaps, you weren't aware of before? That world is how simple it actually is for you to improve your sleep…

The real learning however comes in actioning what you have learnt and making the contents of this book daily and general life habits.

It's for this reason I have created the following "Sleep Action Plans" for you. I really want you to start experimenting with the spirit of this book and if that means starting with small steps, then that's one step closer to you waking up full of energy in the morning and living a lot longer.

I will finish this book the way that I started it, by simply reminding you of what - if you really had to pick just a few great sleep habits, which I hate to do, as there are so many factors (though this book is about keeping it simple for you) - are the absolute winners to take your life to the next level.

Below are the seven key things you would be wise to pay extra attention to in order to wake up every morning bursting full of energy and not feel fed up and frustrated or more importantly STOP WAKING UP TIRED:

1. **Consistency.** Go to bed and wake up at the same time every day.

2. **Eat Early.** Leave at least three hours between food and sleep.

3. **Calm Your Mind.** A busy mind will stop you from sleeping.

4. **Natural Light.** Get this daily as this is key to setting a well-functioning circadian rhythm for you.

5. **Exercise.** Is one of the quickest and easiest ways to make you tired, in turn falling asleep quicker and giving you a deeper sleep.

6. **Stimulants.** Stop consuming caffeine, energy drinks or other stimulants late in the day.

7. **Late Night Liquids.** Fed up with waking up during the night for a loo break which breaks your deep sleep?

My only hope is that having read this workbook you take some action. I would love it if you did it all, as you will feel so much happier and more stable in your emotions on a daily basis, however even if you do just a few things that is amazing and will change your life significantly for the better.

As my job is to help make sleeping well, as easy as possible for readers, I have created two "Action Plans" to help implement the information and advice within this workbook. The first action plan, the next chapter is "the bare bones" giving gentle steps and habits to follow that will enhance your life, without requiring any major life changes. It is my hope that this method will allow you to sleep well and wake up in the morning with a spring in your step.

The following chapter, is then the start of "something special". In this chapter, I build on all that you've read with methods that can greatly maximise your life and will have you "beating your alarm clock" every morning, waking with enthusiasm for the day ahead.

Please note that some aspects will be repeated in both action plans, as this is to save readers from going between the two chapters. Both have a simple to follow plan in place to ensure you get the most out of this workbook as possible.

For those that want that something extra for added energy, please see my website for a whole range of energy, stress and longevity options from one-on-one coaching, courses, corporate workshops and more in-depth research and findings that I purposely didn't include in the workbook to keep it simple and easy to use.

Like most things in life, sleep, energy and living longer is more fun if done with others. This could be with your wife or husband, setting your children up for a great and healthy life, or with your friends to help each other out and point each other in the right direction.

So, without further ado let's get you waking up every morning full of energy and life...!

SLEEP MADE EASY 23

This "action plan" is for those of you who find life works best if you take things slowly but surely and are looking forward to not being woken up during the night.

This is a super easy though still comprehensive list for you to regularly check back in and work through.

This also supports the chapter summaries. However, I have put both in to make it even easier for you, both to focus in on one area and to take a complete overview perspective.

Remove – Things That STOP!! You Sleeping

1. Do you know which chronotype you are, Lion, Bear, Wolf or Dolphin?

2. What time would you like to go to sleep?

3. What time would you like to wake up?

4. Have you set an alarm to go to sleep?

5. Do you get natural daylight for 20 mins in the morning?

6. Are your lights on bright after 7pm in your house?

7. Does your phone, tablet and PC have the blue light filter activated?

8. Are your electronic devices turned off at least an hour before bedtime?

9. Do you have any pains that stop you from sleeping?

10. If so, have you taken any action to find and fix the source?

11. Do you take any medication that interferes with your sleep?

12. If so, have you looked into natural alternatives or other medications?

13. What temperature is your room?

14. Have you installed blackout curtains or blinds?

15. Is your bedroom tidy and free of clutter?

16. Is your bedroom clean?

17. **What time is your last consumption of liquids?**

18. **Is your last coffee or energy drink before midday?**

19. **Is your last meal of the day a clear four hours before bedtime?**

20. **Do you now avoid spicy, sugary and fatty foods after 6pm?**

21. **Have you considered investing in a super king bed to allow you and your partner more space, so not to disturb each other throughout the night?**

22. **Do you have separate duvets?**

23. **Have you got a fan in the bedroom?**

24. **Have you got an air conditioning unit ready for the summer heatwaves?**

25. Do you have people in your life that cause you constant problems?

SUPER SLEEP FOR SUPER PEOPLE 24

This for those of you who really want to take your sleep to the next level, this is a very comprehensive list for you to regularly check back in and work through.

This also supports the chapter summaries; however, I have put both in to make it even easier for you. Both to focus in on one area and to take a complete overview perspective.

Remove – Things That STOP!! You Sleeping

1. Do you know which chronotype you are, Lion, Bear, Wolf or Dolphin?

2. What time would you like to go to sleep?

3. What time would you like to wake up?

4. Have you set an alarm to go to sleep?

5. Do you get natural daylight for 20 mins in the morning?

6. Are your lights on bright after 7pm in your house?

7. Does your phone, tablet and PC have the blue light filter activated?

8. Are your electronic devices turned off at least an hour before bedtime?

9. **Have you bought and actively used your blue blocker glasses?**

10. **Do you have any pains that stop you from sleeping?**

11. **If so, have you taken any action to find and fix the source?**

12. **Do you have regular massages?**

13. **Do you take any medication that interferes with your sleep?**

14. **If so, have you looked into natural alternatives or other medications?**

15. **What temperature is your room?**

16. **Have you installed blackout curtains or blinds?**

17. Is your bedroom tidy and free of clutter?

18. Is your bedroom clean?

19. Do you write down your level of energy every morning?

20. What time is your last consumption of liquids?

21. Is your last coffee before midday?

22. Have you now stopped taking energy drinks?

23. Is your last meal of the day a clear four hours before bedtime?

24. Do you now avoid spicy, sugary and fatty foods after 6pm?

25. Do you sleep in separate bed from your partner on weekdays?

26. If not, have you got a super king bed?

27. Do you have separate duvets?

28. Have you got a fan in the bedroom?

29. Have you got an air conditioning unit ready for the summer heatwaves?

_____

_____

_____

30. Do you have people in your life that cause you constant problems?

_____

_____

_____

Improve – Things That Will Help You Sleep Better

1. **Do you walk most days?**

2. **Do you take a warm shower or bath before bed?**

3. **Have you started meditating?**

4. **Do you exercise most days?**

5. What time do you exercise?

6. What position do you sleep? If on your stomach have you changed this?

7. Have you experimented with pillows between or under your knees?

8. Is your bed made of natural materials?

9. **Is your bed supportive, neither too soft nor too hard?**

10. **Does your bed allow for underneath ventilation?**

FINALLY.... 25

Life is about how you feel and not what you have.

What you have is for the ego and how you feel is for the soul.

There is no better way to live life than feeling good within yourself. Though sleep can't solve all your problems, it's certainly your best starting point in life, to feeling great in yourself every day you arise (well most mornings anyhow).

The second most important thing when it comes to feeling great within yourself, is removing stress and living life full of energy, which is where my next book will take us together...

Thank You for Reading...

Have You Enjoyed This Book?

I really do hope so, and if you have, I would be genuinely grateful for your thoughts and feedback to help improve the book and help others decide if this book is for them.

Please consider leaving a review on Amazon or your favourite store.

HOW RALPH CAN HELP YOU? 26

If you are serious about living life with more energy and less stress all while living longer and making it a key part of your daily life, then there are a few ways Ralph can further help you to achieve your longevity goals.

Depending on your learning style and preferences, Ralph can help you in the following ways:

1. **Corporate Workshops – Onsite Training Programs.**

    If you would like your employees to perform at higher levels, make your business more profitable, all while feeling happier, then the **Sleep for Profit Corporate Workshops** can do this for you.

    It's a one day workshop for ideally 30 of your staff, to show them in quick and simple ways how to sleep better and have a lot more energy every single morning they wake up.

    It's very much focused on building great habits and implementation so that your staff can even start that night and come into work tomorrow feeling better than they ever have!

    We also offer **Stress Mastery Corporate Workshops** for those that have first done the Sleep for Profit Corporate Workshops.

2. **Executive Workshops - Onsite Coaching Programs.**

In addition to your workforce, if you would like a more personalised approach for board members and senior staff, this option is also available.

This is a two-day program, covering everything in Sleep Mastery, plus 1-2-1s at the end of each day with each executive.

This is then also followed up with further coaching calls for each of your executives, to ensure maximum efficiency in the implementation process.

If you understand the power of having well-rested executives that are full of energy and focus, then please get in touch.

3. **Longevity Coaching - Online Coaching Programs.**

Sleep Mastery is a super easy to action, yet comprehensive coaching program for you to master the most important part of longevity...sleep!

Energy Mastery will be released in 2024, which guides you how to reduce stress and have more energy, all while you get more things done and live longer.

To find out more about the above, please visit the website www.thelongevityclinic.co.uk.

WOULD YOU LIKE ANY FURTHER HELP?

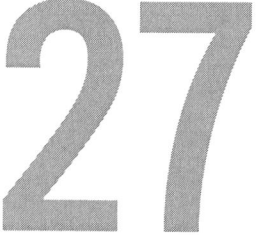

We have a very comprehensive central learning centre on my website, **The Longevity Clinic**, that covers my Longevity Model "RIO – Remove, Improve & Optimise". The link is below.

In addition to my RIO Model on my learning centre, I also have comprehensive articles and guides specific to stress, energy and looking younger.

My website or LinkedIn is the best way to get in touch with me, so please feel free to connect with me on LinkedIn or via the website if there is any way I can help you further.

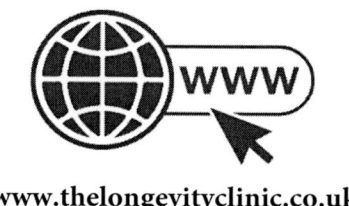

www.thelongevityclinic.co.uk

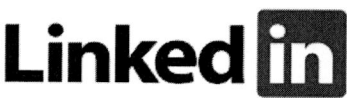

www.linkedin.com/in/ralphwmontague

I have recently, decades later, embraced the world of social media and at long last actually now have an Instagram account!

So please feel free to watch my regular short videos and posts on Instagram. Plus, every week I publish one or two articles on Medium.com with my new perspectives to optimise you and your family for life.

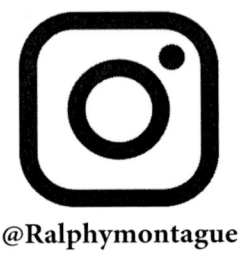

@Ralphymontague

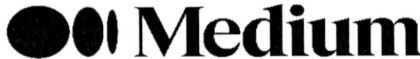

medium.com/@ralphmontague

ABOUT THE AUTHOR
RALPH MONTAGUE

Having been raised in Monmouthshire, before leaving to study at Reading University, where Ralph studied for his Bachelors in investment banking and Master's in commercial property, a career in stock broking was the intended path.

It wasn't long before the urge to do something in the anti-aging world took over his banking and property aspirations.

With Ralph's first anti-aging and aesthetic clinic in 2005, looking and being younger has always been key to Ralph's heart.

Ralph was the founder of The Skin Repair Clinic, a regional chain of aesthetic clinics and previously a director of The Skin Repair Group, a provider of anti-aging and longevity devices such as cryotherapy and hyperbaric oxygen therapy.

He has written numerous books including, the UKs leading aesthetics business book, The Profitable Clinic. Along with STOP!! Killing Yourself...The Beginners Guide to Living Longer. With more to come...

His passion for sleep, stress, energy and longevity evolved from the anti-aging industry he'd been so heavily involved in, which was the basis for The Longevity Clinic. As founding partner the aim of The Longevity Clinic is to educate and guide people in the simplest way possible on how not only can they stop themselves from dying young and before their time, but all while having more energy today and live a healthy and happy life right until the end. With no chronic diseases pestering them for the last decade of their lives.

Ralph certainly practices what he preaches, having a Cryotherapy Chamber, Hyperbaric Oxygen Chamber (HBOT), Oxygen Facial Device, a Skin Repair Pen (micro needling), Fat Freezing Machine, Red Light Therapy, HIFEM Accelerated Muscle Stimulation machine and his most recent addition Adaptive Oxygen Therapy machine (Intermittent Hypoxia), all at home for his personal use and he absolutely loves all these things, using them multiple times a week!

Though no saint, you will still see Ralph out and about getting drunk a few times a year (well a quarter, who am I trying to kid!). Plus, his weekly pizza or curry, and that's the message he wants to spread, you don't have to be perfect and super anal all the time, just most of the time…

Books by the Author

1. STOP!! Killing Yourself…The Beginners Guide to Living Longer.

2. The Profitable Clinic – The Ultimate Guide to Making Money from Owning a Clinic, Spa or High End Beauty Salon!

Future Book Releases

1. STOP!! Stressing Out…The Beginners Guide to More Energy (2023).

2. STOP!! Looking Old…The Beginners Guide to Looking Younger (2024).

INDEX

Night Shift, 37
Noise, 124

O

Onions, 79, 80
Open minded, 28
Optimistic, 28
Organic, 177
Overweight, 8

P

Pain, 7, 42, 44, 48, 50
Paroxetine, 93
Paxil, 94
Pharmacist, 99
Phone, 150
Pillows, 174
Practical, 3, 28
Prazosin, 92
Prednisone, 95
Processed Food, 79
Productivity, 8
Propranolol, 91
Prozac, 94

R

Rapaflo, 93
Rashes, 46
Razadyne, 95
Read, 150
REM, 17, 18, 66, 83, 93, 105
Remove, 7, 21, 33, 44, 119, 212, 220, 237
Right brain, 24
RIO Model, 237
Rivastigmine, 94
Rosuvastatin, 90

S

Sarafem, 94

Sauna, 149
Sertraline, 93
Sheets, 177
Shikfuton, 164
Shower, 150
Side sleeping, 44
Silodosin, 92
Simvastatin, 90
Sleeping position, 44
Socialising, 72
Sotalol, 91
Stable, 28
Statins, 90, 100
Sterapred, 96
Stimulants, 14, 208
Stomach, 195
Stress, 235
Sunburn, 46

T

Tamsulosin, 92
Tatami mat, 164
Technology, 35
Tenormin, 92
Terazosin, 92
The Longevity Clinic, 237, 239
Timolol, 91
Timoptic, 91
Tomatoes, 79, 80
Triamcinolone, 95

U

Uroxatral, 93

V

Ventilation, 160

W

Washing machines, 125

Wolf, 27, 28, 29, 212, 220
Wool, 177

X

Xyzal, 97

Z

LIFE GOT YOU DOWN?
MY NEXT WORKBOOK WAS
WRITTEN FOR YOU…

STOP!!
KILLING
YOURSELF…

THE BEGINNERS LIVING LONGER

AVAILABLE NOW

FEELING STRESSED?
MY NEXT WORKBOOK WAS
WRITTEN FOR YOU...

STOP!!
STRESSING OUT...

THE BEGINNERS GUIDE TO STRESS

COMING IN SPRING 2024